P9-CQZ-011

The Health Robbers

The Health Robbers

How to Protect
Your Money and Your Life

Edited by

STEPHEN BARRETT, M.D.
Chairman, Board of Directors
Lehigh Valley Committee
Against Health Fraud, Inc.

and

GILDA KNIGHT
Executive Assistant,
American Institute of Nutrition

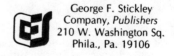
George F. Stickley
Company, *Publishers*
210 W. Washington Sq.
Phila., Pa. 19106

The Health Robbers is a special publication of the Lehigh Valley Committee Against Health Fraud, Inc., an independent organization which was formed in 1969 to combat deception in the field of health. The purposes of the Committee are:

1) To investigate false, deceptive or exaggerated health claims.
2) To conduct a vigorous campaign of public education.
3) To assist appropriate government and consumer-oriented agencies.
4) To bring problems to the attention of lawmakers.

The Lehigh Valley Committee Against Health Fraud is a member organization of the Consumer Federation of America. Since 1970, the Committee has been chartered under the laws of the Commonwealth of Pennsylvania as a not-for-profit corporation. Inquiries about Committee activities may be addressed to P. O. Box 1602, Allentown, Pa. 18105.

Copyright © 1976 The Lehigh Valley Committee Against Health Fraud, Inc.

I.S.B.N. #0-89313-001-X

Library of Congress Catalog Card #76-222-81

All rights reserved under International and Pan-American Copyright Convention. Published in the United States by the George F. Stickley Company, Philadelphia.

INTRODUCTION

Day after day, we hear about our health. Advertisements bombard us. News is sensational. Health books abound.

Unfortunately, much of this information is false.

Health science has never had more to offer than it does today. Yet trust in doctors has fallen . . . and quackery is at an all-time high.

Some exploiters merely want our money. Others, perhaps more confused than crooked, seek converts to their ignorance.

How can we tell experts from pretenders?
How can we get reliable information?
How can we communicate to get better health care from our doctors?

Is our government working or failing to protect us from being cheated?

By exploring these questions, this book should help both your health and your pocketbook.

—THE LEHIGH VALLEY COMMITTEE
AGAINST HEALTH FRAUD, INC.

THIS BOOK IS DEDICATED TO THE TRUTH.
ALL PROFITS FROM ITS SALE RECEIVED BY THE
COMMITTEE WILL BE USED TO FIGHT QUACKERY.

CONTENTS

Contents

FOREWORD

Barnum was right. There's a sucker born every minute. And two to take him. How do I know? Because the victims write to me. And they have been writing to me every day for over 20 years.

Ann Landers receives approximately 7,000 letters a week from readers who represent every conceivable socio-economic group. They live on suburban estates and in the city slums. My correspondents are from 6 to 110 years of age. They are double-dome intellectuals and borderline morons. Almost half of the letters come from men.

Every bag of mail contains at least 150 inquiries that drive me up the wall. "How can they be so stupid?" I ask myself. And then I answer the question. It's not merely stupidity. It's desperation and wishful thinking that wipes out all reason and common sense. I become furious at the exploitation of these good people whose only crime is ignorance and vulnerability.

Here are some examples that crossed my desk just this week:

"Dear Ann: Is it true that musk oil will turn a man on? My husband is 46 years old and sexually dead as a doornail. I've seen this musk oil advertised, but $11 is a lot of money for a little bottle. If you say it will help, I'll buy it."

"Dear Ann: I'm a career girl, 28 years old, and haven't had more than three real dates in my life. The reason is because I am flat-chested. I mean I don't have any bust at all. All my life I've wanted to have nice round bosoms. Please tell me if this cream will help. (Advertisement enclosed.) As you can see, the 'before' and 'after' pictures are very convincing. What do you say?"

Foreword

"Dear Ann: Is it true that cooking in aluminum will cause cancer? A man came to the door yesterday selling cookware. He scared the life out of me. His utensils cost $450 for the complete set. If what he says is true, about cancer, I mean, it sure would be worth it. But I hate to throw out these perfectly good pots and pans I've used for 10 years."

One after another the letters come—from the "exotic dancer" who wants to grow "georgeous nails in 20 days"—from the overweight housewife who will do *anything* to get thin except quit eating the things she loves. Then there are the females with bags under their eyes and extra chins who are sure they will look ten years younger if they use the enriched cream (secret formula) for thirty days. The trouble is—it's awfully expensive. "But it would be well worth the money if it works," writes Mrs. W. from Sheboygan. "Cheaper than a face lift. And no pain."

When men write and ask if the pomade and treatments guaranteed to grow hair will help, I often reply, "Yes. It will help the manufacturer and the man who sells it. They will get rich. As for you, it will help flatten your wallet, but it won't do anything for your bald head."

The letters from teenagers are especially pathetic. "My skin is such a mess of pimples and blackheads no girl would go out with me, so I don't even ask. Please don't suggest a doctor. I can't afford one. This soap and cream combination promises results within ten days. What do you think, Ann? And while I'm at it, Ann, maybe you can tell me if this mail-order speech course will help my brother. He stutters. His grades are awful. He's not dumb, he's just ashamed to speak up in class."

"Dear Ann: Our sex life is blah after 15 years. My husband wants to try a sex clinic, but some friends of ours went and you wouldn't believe the things they were asked to do. I don't go for that far-out stuff like changing partners. Frankly, I'm scared. What do you think?"

Foreword

The saddest letters of all come from relatives of the desperately ill, those who are dying of cancer, or kidney disease. "Our family doctor said there was nothing more he could do, so we took mom to this wonderful chiropractor. She seems a little stronger today. Do you think, Ann, that we should have brought her to the chiropractor from the beginning and not wasted all that time and money on a specialist with a fancy diploma from Harvard hanging on his office wall?"

Every letter gets a personal reply in the mail, if there's a name and an address. I urge my readers to beware of quacks and phonies. I warn them against the charlatans and fakers. More often than I care to admit, I have received in return a seething reply: "How dare you take away our hope! I'll bet you are on the payroll of the American Medical Association. The medical doctor didn't do anything but send us big bills. Jesus Christ is the greatest healer of them all. Now that we have put our child in His hands, we know everything is going to be all right."

How can the public be protected against phonies, quacks, and unscrupulous money-grubbers who prey on the insecure, the frightened, and the sick? The answer is education. And that is what this book is all about.

Each chapter is written by a highly respected authority in his or her field. In the pages that follow, you will read the truth about a wide variety of food fads, worthless gadgets, sex clinics, and organized "health plans" designed to separate fools from their money. Ignorance is NOT bliss—and it never will be. Only the truth can set you free.

Ann Landers

About the Contributors

Philip R. Alper, M.D., who practices internal medicine and endocrinology, is Assistant Clinical Professor of Medicine at the University of California Medical Center in San Francisco. He is editor of the *California Society of Internal Medicine Newsletter* and a contributing editor to *Medical Economics* magazine.

Sidney L. Arje, M.D., is Vice-President for Professional Development of the American Cancer Society. A specialist in obstetrics and gynecology, he has been chief of the obstetrics-gynecology service at several U.S. Naval installations and was Commanding Officer of the U.S. Naval Hospital in St. Albans, N.Y.

Stephen Barrett, M.D., a practicing psychiatrist, is the nation's most vigorous opponent of health quackery. Since 1970, he has been Chairman of the Board of Directors of the Lehigh Valley Committee Against Health Fraud, Inc. He is also a member of the Committee on Quackery of the Pennsylvania Medical Society and has been a member of the Committee on Health Fraud of the Pennsylvania Health Council.

Irene L. Bartlett, an entomologist, has spent 20 years collecting and writing information on unproven methods of cancer treatment. She is the author of "Unproven Methods of Cancer Treatment" published by the American Cancer Society in 1966, 1967 and a revised edition in 1971.

Diana Benzaia is Associate Director of Public Information for The Arthritis Foundation and specializes in public health education and community action. She has also worked for The National Foundation/March of Dimes.

Mary Bernhardt is Secretary of the American Dental Association's Council on Dental Health which includes community fluoridation in its consideration of preventive dentistry and public health.

Robert C. Derbyshire, M.D., a practicing surgeon, is a leading authority on the licensing and discipline of physicians. He serves as Secretary-Treasurer of the New Mexico Board of Medical Examiners and is Past-President of the Federation of State Medical Boards of the United States.

H. William Gross, D.D.S., a practicing dentist and a dental adviser to Pennsylvania Blue Shield, has been particularly active in promoting fluoridation on behalf of organized dentistry. He is President of the Lehigh Valley Committee Against Health Fraud, Inc., Public Health Chairman of the Lehigh Valley Dental Society and Chairman of the Governmental Relations Committee of the Second District of the Pennsylvania Dental Association.

Max Gunther, a former staff member of TIME Magazine, is now a freelance journalist.

Victor Herbert, M.D., J.D., is a specialist in both internal medicine and nutrition and is also an attorney. A leading research scientist, he is medical investigator and Director

About the Contributors

of the Hematology and Nutrition Unit of the Bronx VA Hospital. He holds professorships in both medicine and pathology at Columbia College of Physicians and Surgeons.

Wallace F. Janssen, former Director of Public Information for the U.S. Food and Drug Administration, was responsible for the public warning which saved more than 6,000 people from being victimized by the Hoxsey cancer treatment. He was also an originator of the National Congresses on Quackery, and is now FDA Historian.

William T. Jarvis, Ph.D., a consumer health specialist, is Associate Professor of Preventive and Community Dentistry at the Loma Linda University School of Dentistry. His teaching areas cover research methods, nutrition, public health, health fraud and dental ethics.

Thomas H. Jukes, Ph.D., is Professor of Medical Physics and Lecturer in Nutrition at the University of California in Berkeley. A distinguished biochemist, Dr. Jukes has done nutritional research for many years. He is a vigorous opponent of nutritional quackery and has been active in the formation of the Northern California Council Against Health Fraud.

Murray Katz, M.D.C.M., is a practicing physician in Montreal, Canada. He is consultant on health matters to the Quebec Division of the Consumer Association of Canada and the Quebec Committee Against Health Fraud, Inc.

Reverend Lester Kinsolving, an Episcopal worker-priest, is a religion columnist and White House Correspondent for the National News Syndicate, and an editorial commentator and investigative reporter for radio station WAVA in Washington, D.C. He has been nominated for the Pulitzer Prize by the *San Francisco Chronicle* and the *San Francisco Examiner*.

Gilda Knight, Executive Assistant for the American Institute of Nutrition since 1965, is also managing editor of *AIN Nutrition Notes*.

William H. Masters, M.D., began his medical career as an obstetrician-gynecologist. In the late 1960's, he attained national prominence when he and Virginia E. Johnson published the book *Human Sexual Response*. He is Director of the Reproductive Biology Research Foundation, a center for treating couples with sexual difficulties and for training sex therapists.

Jean Mayer, Ph.D., Sc.D., chaired the White House Conference on Nutrition and Health in 1969 and has served on a number of United Nations committees on nutrition requirements. He is a syndicated nutrition columnist and has written several books (his latest is *A Diet for Living*). After many years as Professor of Nutrition at the Harvard University School of Public Health, Dr. Mayer recently became President of Tufts University.

Jacob Nevyas, Ph.D., Sc.D., for almost 40 years a teacher of biochemistry at the Pennsylvania College of Optometry, lectures and is an editor of papers and textbooks on scientific subjects.

Lois V. Smith served until recently as Program Associate for the American Cancer Society's Section on Unproven Methods of Cancer Management. Previously she was Executive Medical Secretary and Research Assistant at the Sloan-Kettering Institute for Cancer Research in New York.

About the Contributors

Bob Sprague is a newspaper reporter and freelance writer who currently works for *The Free Press* of Quakertown, Pa. Raised in a fluoridated community, he got his first cavity at the age of 32.

Arthur Taub, M.D., Ph.D., is a neurologist whose subspecialty is the diagnosis and treatment of pain. He is Clinical Professor of Anesthesiology. Lecturer in Neurology, and Director of the Section for the Study and Treatment of Pain, Department of Anesthesiology, Yale University School of Medicine.

James Harvey Young, Ph.D., Professor of History at Emory University, is a social historian who has a particular interest in the development of food and drug regulation in America. He has been a member of the National Advisory Food and Drug Council to the U.S. Food and Drug Administration. His books, *The Toadstool Millionaires* and *The Medical Messiahs*, trace history of health quackery in America and efforts to control it.

ACKNOWLEDGMENTS

Chapter 6 is adapted from *The Medical Impostor*, a chapter in *Medical Licensure and Discipline in the United States*, written by Dr. Robert Derbyshire and published by the Johns Hopkins University Press. It appears in this book with the kind permission of the author and publisher.

Chapter 7 is reprinted from the November 1974 issue of *Today's Health* with the kind permission of the American Medical Association, Dr. William Masters, and Max Gunther who collaborated with Dr. Masters in its preparation.

Portions of Chapter 12 are reproduced from *Americans Love Hogwash* with the kind permission of the author, Dr. Edward Rynearson, Emeritus Professor of Medicine, The Mayo Clinic.

Chapter 23 is adapted from *The Persistence of Medical Quackery in America* by Dr. James Harvey Young, and appears with the kind permission of *American Scientist*, journal of Sigma Xi, The Scientific Research Society of North America.

Permission to use the following illustrations is gratefully acknowledged: Page 98—Leonard Herman; page 170—King Features Syndicate; page 316—Al Kaufman and *Resident and Staff Physician;* page 326—*American Medical News.*

The Committee wishes to thank Joseph Botta and Ralpha Senderowitz for their many helpful suggestions in the preparation of this manuscript.

PART ONE
Health Robbers and How to Spot Them

THE CRUELLEST KILLERS

Cancer quackery is big business, with an estimated yearly income in the billions. It is also cruel business, for its customers come in desperate fear. Those customers who come while also undergoing good medical care will buy only empty promises. But those . . . who delay or abandon medicine's best, will purchase death.

BY

SIDNEY L. ARJE, M.D.
Vice-President for Professional Development
and
LOIS V. SMITH
Ex-Program Associate, Unproven Methods
The American Cancer Society

John Miner was deeply shaken by what he saw:

"The right side of her face was that of an angel. The left half was covered with a growth so monstrous as to seem beyond nature's capacity to be cruel and grotesque . . . When I walked out of her room, I knew two things: Linda Epping would soon die; second, when it happened, I would seek a murder indictment."

When Miner made this report, he was Assistant District Attorney for Los Angeles County. The case had started routinely in 1961 with a complaint from Linda's parents. One Marvin Phillips had bilked them out of $739 by falsely promising to cure their eight-year old daughter of cancer of the eye.

Linda had been scheduled for surgery which would remove her left eye and surrounding tissues. Cure was possible, her doctors thought, because the tumor did not appear to have spread. But shortly before the operation could be performed, a fateful conversation took place. In the hospital waiting room, Linda's distraught parents met a couple named Eaton. According to Mrs. Eaton, a chiropractor named Marvin Phillips had cured their son's brain tumor without using surgery.

Her hopes aroused, Mrs. Epping telephoned Dr. Phillips and informed him of Linda's diagnosis. Without even seeing the child, Phillips replied, "Yes, absolutely," he could help by "chemically balancing" her body.

Elated by this promise, the Eppings removed Linda from the hospital and took her to Phillips for treatment with vitamins, food supplements and laxatives (up to 124 pills plus 150 drops of iodine solution daily). In addition, Phillips "adjusted" Linda's spine at his office and told the Eppings to manipulate the ball of her foot each day until she cried.

Despite the new "treatment," the tumor grew

2

quickly. Within three weeks, it was tennis-ball size and had pushed Linda's eye out of its socket. There was no longer any hope that surgery could save her. She died within a few months.

Phillips was subsequently convicted of second degree murder and sentenced to prison.

Promoters of Unproven Methods

Cancer quackery is big business, with an estimated yearly income in the billions. It is also cruel business, for its customers come in desperate fear. Those customers who come while also undergoing good medical care will buy only empty promises. But those like the Eppings, who delay or abandon medicine's best, will purchase death.

Promoters of quackery are often closely attuned to the emotions of their customers. They may exude warmth, interest, friendliness, enthusiasm and compassion. Most important, they assure their frightened patients that they will be helped.

Unfortunately, recognizing quackery is not always easy. Its promoters may present a very professional appearance. They may wear white coats and use scientific-sounding words. They may use the title "Doctor" and display a variety of elaborately framed diplomas. Close investigation might reveal that their credentials come from "diploma mills" which have no recognized academic standing. Degrees such as "N.D." (Doctor of Naturopathy), "Ph.N." (Philosopher of Naturopathy) and "Ms.D." (Doctor of Metaphysics) are in this category. It is important to realize, however, that a few promoters of unproven methods are highly educated scientists who have strayed from their fields of competency.

Andrew C. Ivy, M.D., Ph.D., is an example of the latter. Dr. Ivy was highly respected by the scientific world for his contributions to medicine. But in 1959 he withdrew from the established medical community and became interested in "Krebiozen." This substance is derived from horses which have been injected with a sterile extract of Actinomyces, the fungus which causes "lumpy jaw" in cattle. The original substance was developed and brought to Dr. Ivy's attention by Dr. Steven Durovic, a Yugoslavian physician. The two doctors claimed it gave fantastic results in the treatment of cancer patients. But in 1963, 24 cancer specialists reviewed the medical records of 504 Krebiozen patients which had been submitted to the National Cancer Institute. Their conclusion, after thorough study, was that Krebiozen did not work against cancer in humans.

In 1965, court action brought by the Food and Drug Administration banned interstate shipment of Krebiozen. No longer associated with Dr. Durovic, Dr. Ivy is now concerned with a drug which he calls "Carcalon." It has been determined, however, that Carcalon is merely another name for Krebiozen.

Recognizing Quackery

Quacks tend to be isolated from established scientific facilities and associations. They do not report their results in scientific journals. Instead they rely on publication in the free press and other non-medical channels. Often their cure is "secret" or bears their own name. They claim persecution by the medical profession or government agencies. They keep scanty records or no records at all.

Quacks rely heavily on stories of people they have supposedly cured. But such evidence is not reliable. Many cancer patients have given testimonials, believing they have been cured, only to find out later that they still have the disease. Others did not have cancer to begin with. They only thought they did. Some satisfied

4

customers are patients who used unproven methods together with good medical care. Charmed by the quack, however, they believe that his treatment is what helped them. Although spontaneous remissions of cancer are rare, they do occur. Thus it is possible, though unlikely, that someone who uses an unproven method could have a spontaneous remission at the same time.

To be classified as effective or proven, a treatment method must meet certain standards. Patients who are treated with a particular method must do better than similar patients who do not receive that treatment. Proof that the patients actually had cancer must be available in the form of specimens which can be examined by microscope. Patients must be followed for many years to measure the true outcome of their cases, and the number of patients must be large enough to rule out chance as a factor. Experiments which are valid can be repeated and thus confirmed by the scientific community.

Unproven Methods

Cancer quackery is as old as recorded history and probably has existed since cancer was recognized as a disease. Thousands of worthless folk remedies, diets, drugs, devices and procedures have been promoted for cancer management.

—*Corrosive agents* have been applied directly to tumors with the hope of burning them away. Turpentine is an old favorite, having been used by quacks since ancient times. In recent years, scientists have found chemicals which can destroy very superficial skin cancers. Except for that, however, corrosive agents are worthless.

—Other popular *folk remedies* include red clover tea, salves made from zinc chloride and blood root, plant material sun-dried in pewter, and even "live green frogs applied to external cancer till they die." Plants said to be used by Indians to shrink heads have been promoted—with the theory that if they could shrink heads, they could shrink cancer.

Beginning in 1922, a naturopath named Harry M. Hoxsey amassed a fortune treating cancer patients with worthless folk remedies. He used a combination of internal and external substances. The internal medicine, taken by mouth, was prescribed "in all cases" to "restore the body to physiological normalcy." It contained potassium iodide and such things as red clover, licorice, burdock root, Stillingia root, Berberis root, poke root, cascara, prickly ash bark and buckthorn bark. Hoxsey's external medicines contained corrosive agents such as arsenic sulfide.

Between 1950 and 1960, vigorous action by the Food and Drug Administration drove Hoxsey out of business. His methods, however, are still advocated by health food stores.

—*Diets* are another way to "remedy" cancer. The usual theory behind them is that cancer is caused by an "imbalance" in the body or by accumulated "poisons" or "impurities." Proper diet would then "detoxify" the body. One such regimen is promoted by Johanna Brandt, N.D., in her book *The Grape Cure*. The patient must eat one-half pound of any "good variety of grapes," starting at 8 A.M. and repeating every two hours, for seven meals a day. For one or two weeks, nothing else may be added except for water. Then sour milk, raw vegetables, salads, dried fruits, nuts, honey, olive oil and certain fresh fruits may be eaten. Neither the Grape Cure nor any other special diet has any value in the prevention or treatment of cancer.

—Useless *biological products* used to treat cancer include vaccines and preparations derived from the patient's own blood and/or urine or from animal blood

6

and/or urine. One such vaccine was the "Radio-Sulpho Cancer Cure" which originated in Denver, Colorado. Philip Schuch, Jr., President of the Radio-Sulpho Company, claimed he could "culture cancer germs direct from the cancer vaccine" he discovered. Although he was not a physician, he called himself a "cancer specialist." His treatment consisted of washing the cancer with Radio-Sulfo Brew, applying a Limburger cheese "poultice," and repeating every twelve hours. However, "to stand the powerful drawing power of the cheese," Schuch warned, "a person must be strong and healthy."

—Worthless *diagnostic testing* is another fertile field for quackery. One such worthless test was developed by Dr. H. H. Beard, a biochemist. Beard claimed that by measuring a sex hormone in your urine, he could detect cancer in your body within two to three weeks after it started. His book, *A New Approach to Conquering Cancer, Rheumatic Fever and Heart Disease,* contains a chapter on preventing malignancy by using his "Beard Anthrone Test." Advertisements for the book included instructions for collecting specimens which could be mailed to Dr. Beard in Fort Worth, Texas.

In 1965 the California Cancer Advisory Council and the Department of Public Health studied the Beard Anthrone Test and found it useless in the detection of cancer in humans. In May 1967, Beard was indicted by a Federal Grand Jury for mail fraud. Pleading "no contest," he received a six-month suspended sentence and one year probation. But before the court had halted his activities, Beard had conducted an estimated 15,000 tests for which he had received approximately $150,000.

—Through the years, hundreds of worthless *drugs* have been promoted for cancer prevention or cure. "Laetrile" heads today's list of all forms of cancer quackery. Laetrile contains the chemical amygdalin, a substance which is abundant in the kernels of peaches, apricots, bitter almonds and apple seeds. Such seeds are dangerous to eat because amygdalin breaks down into a toxic cyanide. Laetrile is sometimes referred to as "vitamin B-17." (There is no medically or nutritionally recognized vitamin B-17.)

Although Laetrile has been used for more than 25 years, there is no scientific evidence that it is safe or effective. In 1953 the Cancer Commission of the California Medical Society published information on 44 cancer patients who had been treated with Laetrile during the previous year. Nineteen had died of their disease and there was no evidence that Laetrile had helped any of the others.

Laetrile's backers have not been able to prove that it can control cancer in animals. Many independent laboratory experiments have also been negative. Without such proof, it is illegal for the drug to be used to treat humans in this country. Unfortunately, international trafficking of Laetrile has become big business. The United States Customs Service estimates that 20 to 25 distributors are involved in a network which encompasses Mexico, Canada and Germany. Laetrile which is smuggled into the United States costs as much as $50 for a half-ounce vial for injection. Tablets, which cost about three cents to make, sell for nearly two dollars in the U.S.

Backers of Laetrile

Ernesto Contreras, M.D., a licensed physician in Tijuana, Mexico, operates a hospital and "cancer clinic." It is estimated that more than 5,000 Americans have paid more than $4,000,000 for his Laetrile treatment.

The International Association of Cancer Victims and

Friends (IACVF) was formed in 1963 to "restore the cancer victim's life and free choice of treatment and doctor." The Association's founder, Cecile Pollack Hoffman, was a San Diego schoolteacher who underwent a radical mastectomy for breast cancer in 1959. In 1962, she had further surgery due to the spread of the cancer. Her husband, while sitting in an airport waiting room, happened to pick up a paperback book entitled *Laetrile: Control for Cancer* by Glenn D. Kittler.

After reading the book, Mrs. Hoffman sought further information. Not long afterward, she became a staunch supporter of Laetrile and developed a belief that it had saved her life. Although she died of metastatic cancer in July 1969, her organization has continued to operate. In 1975 it claimed to have 25 chapters and a membership of "thousands."

IACVF sponsors conventions at which unproven cancer remedies are promoted and sometimes sold. It distributes information on the availability of unproven cancer remedies and makes arrangements for travel to Mexico for treatment. IACVF members, who pay dues according to membership category, receive the *Cancer News Journal* which contains many misleading articles about unproven cancer treatments. Dr. Contreras is a "Life Member" of IACVF.

The Cancer Control Society was formed in 1973 in Los Angeles by dissident members of the IACVF after disputes over major policy and the distribution of the proceeds of book sales. The new group favors aggressive lobbying and court action against government restrictions on unproven remedies of every kind. It is working toward national organization.

The Committee for Freedom of Choice in Cancer Therapy, Inc., was founded in 1972 by Robert Bradford, a Stanford University physicist. This group was able to establish large numbers of local chapters throughout the United States within a matter of months. Its interests appear to be political rather than medical, with emphasis on Constitutional rights and freedoms. Persons affiliated with this Committee appear also to be closely linked to "underground railroads" which provide access to those who provide unproven remedies. Some bookshops associated with the John Birch Society have served as meeting places for the Committee and as sources of literature about unproven treatments. The Committee has made wide distribution of a one-hour film called *World Without Cancer* as well as a book of the same name. In December 1975, Robert Bradford was arrested by a U.S. Customs agent on a charge of smuggling Laetrile into the United States. As this book goes to press, he is awaiting trial in a federal court.

The National Health Federation (NHF) is another membership organization which promotes the gamut of questionable health theories and practices. Many of its leaders have been in serious legal difficulty (see Chapter 13). Since its founding in 1955, it has been fighting vigorously against government regulation of unproven methods. Its legal defense fund assists those who are being prosecuted for sale of unproven cancer remedies. Its main impact, however, is its ability to generate huge amounts of mail to Congress and other agencies. In 1957 an NHF campaign resulted in 200,000 communications to the FDA to protest its interference with the Hoxsey cancer treatment. More recently, FDA efforts for more honest labeling of nutrition products triggered an avalanche of NHF-inspired mail. During the past four years, an estimated 2,000,000 letters have urged Congress to limit government regulation of food supplements. NHF-supported legislation to do this could make many unproven cancer remedies freely available.

Promotion Through the Media

Freedom of the press is an important factor in the promotion of unproven cancer remedies. Books, especially if they are on so-called "controversial" medical problems, are quite appealing to the public. Many books about unproven remedies are cleverly written so that the reader may think he is getting valuable information when he is not. Some examples are *The Incredible Story of Krebiozen: A Matter of Life and Death; Vitamin B-17: Forbidden Weapon Against Cancer;* and *Has Dr. Max Gerson A True Cancer Cure?*

Entertainers, socially prominent persons and other celebrities are often called upon to promote unproven methods. These individuals, while often sincere, do not have the scientific background to judge the value of the method they are promoting. Cancer quackery gets additional support from sensational mass circulation newspapers and magazines and from radio and television talk shows. A number of so-called "health" magazines which are especially interested in unproven treatment regimens publish articles on the latest "theories" and "advances" in cancer management. Examples of these are the National Health Federation *Bulletin* (circulation 18,500), the *Herald of Health* (circulation 4,000), and *Prevention* (circulation 1,600,000).

Proponents of "freedom of choice" in cancer therapy often demand to know why drugs which do not cause direct harm should be banned from use in the United States. After all, they say, might they not do some good? The answer to this argument is that the laws which ban unproven cancer remedies are essential to protect the public from all worthless remedies. The psychological "benefit" of worthless remedies in apparently hopeless cases is far outweighed by the disastrous results of using such products *instead* of effective treatment. Our society should not allow the pockets of those who make false claims to be lined by the unfortunates who fall for such claims.

Role of the American Cancer Society

In 1955, the American Cancer Society began a program to help fight cancer quackery. At that time, there was little factual information concerning this problem and there were no state laws to combat it.

A Committee on Unproven Methods of Cancer Management was formed to serve as a central coordinating force in this field. The Committee is concerned with public and professional education as well as legal matters. Its membership includes experts in these fields. The Committee has issued many reports on individual unproven cancer remedies and tests. Its "State Model Cancer Act," modeled after the California anti-quackery act, has encouraged passage of laws against cancer quackery in nine states (Colorado, Illinois, Kentucky, Maryland, Nevada, North Dakota, Ohio and Pennsylvania).

The National Office of the American Cancer Society has established an information clearinghouse which contains the world's largest collection of information about cancer quackery. Material from its files is used to answer thousands of inquiries from health professionals, writers and the general public. Information about unproven methods is also published in *Ca—A Cancer Journal for Clinicians* which is distributed, free of charge, to more than 360,000 physicians and medical students in the United States.

The Cruellest Killers

Most cancer patients can be cured if treated properly and in time. One and one-half million Americans are alive today because their cancers were cured by prompt use of *proven* methods of surgery, radiation or chemotherapy.

You might think that as medical treatment has become more effective, quackery would diminish in proportion. That has not happened. Modern communication and our free press have enabled unproven methods to get enormous publicity—luring many unsuspecting Americans to try them.

Many people who promote unproven methods of cancer management are well-meaning individuals who are sincere in their beliefs. The rest are profiteers. Regardless of their motivation, however, one thing is clear. Incurable cancer patients who waste their life's savings on false hopes, and potentially curable patients who die from delay of proper treatment, are victims of quackery at its cruellest.

Recommended Reading

The Victimizing of Desperate Cancer Patients, by Terri Schultz and Bard Lindeman, *Today's Health,* November 1973.

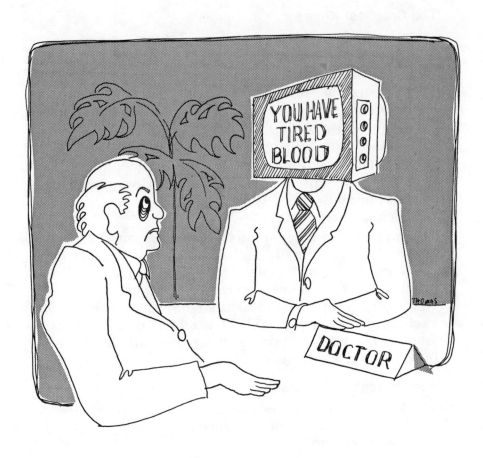

THE PILL PEDDLERS

"The desire to take medicine is perhaps the greatest feature which distinguishes man from animals."

—Sir William Osler

"Advertising should be free of statements, illustrations or implications which are offensive to good taste, and should not distort or exaggerate facts as to size, appearance, effect or usage."

From the Code of Advertising Practices of the Proprietary Association, 1972

BY

MURRAY S. KATZ, M.D.C.M.
Consultant on Health Affairs
Quebec Division
Consumer Association of Canada

Suppose you buy a car and when you try to drive off the dealer's lot, you find it won't start. Looking under the hood, you discover it has no engine. You would call this a fraud and would not accept it. Yet throughout North America, buyers of many patent (non-prescription) medicines are getting the equivalent of cars without engines—such products as cough medicines which contain no effective anti-cough ingredients, sleeping pills which contain no sedatives, and "germ-killers" which do not kill enough germs to be helpful. When you buy a car that has no engine, the fraud is easy to discover. But buyers of patent medicines have no simple way to tell whether they are being cheated.

Used properly, patent medicines can relieve the symptoms of certain ailments. (Patent medicines are also called "over-the-counter" or "OTC" drugs.) Used properly, they can avoid the time and cost of unnecessary visits to a doctor. But the scientific facts are clear. The vast majority of non-prescription medicines do not deserve the credit the public gives them.

Consider mouthwashes, for example. There are more than one hundred varieties on the market. People tend to buy them for three reasons: to make their breath smell better, to clean their teeth, or to treat colds and sore throats. Yet mouthwashes cannot do any of these things effectively.

A major cause of bad breath is food which is decaying between and on the surfaces of the teeth. Mouthwashes generally do smell good and leave a scented odor in your mouth (for a few minutes) which could mislead you into thinking that your mouth is clean. But there are no shortcuts to good oral hygiene. Rinsing your mouth with mouthwash cannot remove food particles as effectively as proper brushing. Nor is a mouthwash more effective than plain water. Good oral hygiene should also include the use of dental floss to clean out

16

areas of plaque which contain harmful bacteria which produce tooth decay. Bad breath can also be caused by what you eat. Alcohol, as well as aromatic foodstuffs like garlic and onions, can cause unpleasant breath odors which actually come from your lungs. Here again, any effect which mouthwash has in masking such odors is likely to last only a few minutes.

*Isodyne** mouthwash advertises that it can "stop sore throat pain" and "reduce inflammation." These claims may be true in the sense that rinsing the mouth with a liquid may relieve sore throat symptoms temporarily. But rinsing with mouthwash is no more effective than rinsing with warm water. *Listerine* advertising has been more misleading. By claiming that *Listerine* "kills germs on contact," it suggests that the product exerts a curative effect. It is true that mouthwashes can kill some germs on contact, but this will not prevent or alter the course of an infection. Germs in the tiny crevices in the mouth and within infected tissues cannot be reached or washed out. Germs which are washed off the surface of infected areas quickly grow back.

Some mouthwashes have a high alcohol content which can cause excessive drying of the mouth. But a more subtle danger exists for mouthwash users. The claims of germ-killing may mislead people into thinking that mouthwash is a sensible treatment for a cold or sore throat. Many people feel safe in treating themselves with a mouthwash and then consulting a doctor if they don't improve. Is there any harm in that? Yes, there can be. The decision about consulting a doctor should be based on more scientific grounds.

---

* Author's note: I do not mean to imply that products named in this chapter are the only (or the worst) offenders in their product groups. I have simply selected examples with which readers are likely to be familiar.

Managing Your Own "Cold"

If you decide to treat your cold by yourself, your first step should be a preliminary survey. Do you have a fever? A skin rash? An earache? A sore throat? Do you feel well enough to carry out your usual activities for that day? Or do you feel "lousy" or "really sick"?

If you have an earache, there is likely to be a bacterial infection present. This requires a visit to your doctor. Don't put any patent medicine drops in your ear. They won't cure you and may only make examination by the doctor more difficult. If the doctor determines that you have a bacterial infection, he will prescribe an antibiotic. Don't try to treat an earache with the so-called "decongestants" of cough and cold medications. They won't get rid of the infection.

If you have a fever, you might decide to use aspirin or acetaminophen. One brand is as good as another—so buy the cheapest. The correct dose of either for adults is two five-grain tablets every four to six hours. As a general rule, if a fever lasts more than 48 hours, it's time to consult a doctor.

Some people find that sore throats can be relieved by gargling which helps to break up dried mucus crusts at the back of the throat. Salt water (one-half teaspoon of salt dissolved in a glass of warm water) is an inexpensive preparation. Don't waste your money on mouthwash. If you have a sore throat and feel "lousy," that is reason to consult a doctor. Sore throats caused by the streptococcus bacterium should be treated with an antibiotic. Left untreated, a small percentage of "strep throats" will lead to rheumatic fever or glomerulonephritis (a kidney disease). Your doctor can diagnose a strep throat by means of a throat culture.

If your nose is blocked, you may be tempted to seek relief with decongestant nosedrops or nasal sprays. You should do so with great caution. *Use of these products can lead to "rebound" congestion—actual worsening of the congestion caused by too frequent use.* Rebound can be a worse problem than the original reason for using the decongestant. So nosedrops or nasal sprays should be used only when absolutely necessary, at most two or three times a day. You might, for example, decide to use one at bedtime so that your stopped nose does not keep you from sleeping. The best type of nasal decongestant is one that contains a single "vaso-constrictor" drug such as phenylephrine hydrochloride. Decongestants may relieve a clogged nose when taken by mouth in high enough dose. But such dosage can also cause nervousness, dizziness, insomnia and a rise of blood pressure. Some products sold without a prescription (*Contac*, for example) contain a decongestant or other ingredients in so-called "sustained" release form—meant to give "twelve-hour relief." Such preparations tend to be erratic, however.

The North American public spends close to one billion dollars per year for so-called cough or cold remedies. These usually contain two or more of the following ingredients:

1) A pain reliever such as aspirin. Much of the relief which people get from cold remedies is the result of the aspirin they contain. But many aspirin-containing products do not provide the best amount of aspirin to help you. The simplest and least expensive way to get the proper dosage of aspirin is to use ordinary aspirin tablets.

2) A nasal decongestant such as phenylephrine or phenylpropanolamine.

3) An anti-cough agent such as dextromethorphan or codeine sulfate. By interfering with your cough reflex, these drugs can be useful in controlling a dry, hacking

cough. The dosage of dextromethorphan is 10 milligrams three times a day. The dosage of codeine sulfate is 10 milligrams every four to six hours, but in many states, codeine cannot be purchased without a prescription. Sucking on hard candy, drinking warm liquids, and using a vaporizer may also be effective. If these measures are not successful in relieving a dry, hacking cough within 48 hours, your next step should be in the direction of your doctor. Cough suppressants should not be used for *productive* (phlegm-producing) coughs without a doctor's advice—for it may be important to allow your lungs to clear themselves by coughing up secretions.

4) An expectorant such as ammonium salts, glycerol guaiacolate (guaifenesin) or syrup of ipecac. These ingredients are supposed to help you cough up thick mucus from your lungs. But their effectiveness is questionable. In some cases they merely increase the amount of secretions present—making it harder for your lungs to clear themselves. The best way to help loosen secretions in your lungs is to drink plenty of liquids.

Some cough medicines combine expectorants with cough suppressants. This is questionable because these ingredients may work against each other.

5) An antihistamine such as chlorpheniramine or methapyrilene. These drugs tend to dry the membranes of the nose and throat. They are primarily effective against cold-like symptoms caused by allergies. Antihistamines can cause drowsiness, a potentially dangerous side effect. If you think you have symptoms caused by an allergy, ask your doctor which antihistamine to use.

Over the years, most cough and cold remedies have been irrational mixtures of ingredients. Many have contained substances which do nothing to help you.

Some contained potentially useful drugs, but not in high enough amounts to be effective. And some contained ingredients which are potentially dangerous or which work against each other. Currently, many cough and cold remedies are being reformulated in response to the product review being conducted by the FDA (described later in this chapter). Judging the outcome of this review process will take several years. In the meantime, your basic policy should be to use products which contain only one active ingredient. For most colds, plenty of fluids—plus aspirin (or acetaminophen) for aches, pains or fever—will be all you need.

Many people treat the aches and pains which accompany a cold with camphor-containing products. Among the favorites are *Vicks VapoRub, Camphor Spirits, Menard's Liniment, Ben-Gay Children's Rub, Camphorated Oil* and *Sloan's Liniment.* Camphor's pleasant aroma leads people to think it is good for them.

When rubbed on the skin, camphor causes redness because of its irritating properties. It can also have a local anesthetic effect, causing numbness of the skin and mucous membranes. When inhaled, camphor gives a cooling sensation. What actually takes place, however, is that nerve endings in the nose which are sensitive to cold are stimulated.

Does all of this do any good? Available evidence shows that camphorated products have no beneficial effect upon the duration or symptoms of a cold and may sometimes be harmful. Covering the skin with a camphor-containing product may give a pleasant, warm feeling. But it also may interfere with the body's ability to lower a fever. Camphor's penetrating odor may give the impression that it is opening clogged nasal or bronchial passages. But far from clearing your respiratory passages, its vapors actually irritate them more. You can experience this for yourself by holding

21

an open bottle of a camphor product near your nose. After a few minutes, your eyes will start to tear and you may even have to cough.

Camphor products are highly poisonous when eaten. Each year, hundreds of curious children and careless adults are poisoned (some fatally) by accidental consumption of these products.

Consumer Psychology

If you were buying a car, many factors might influence your selection. But if it couldn't run, you wouldn't want it. With patent medicines, however, consumer satisfaction does not necessarily require the presence of effective ingredients. There are two reasons for this. The first is that most illnesses are self-limited. The second is a matter of psychology.

When people feel better after taking a medication, they tend to think that the medication has helped them. But to *really* determine whether a medication is effective, it is necessary to know whether the improvement is caused by the medicine or would have happened just the same without it. Scientists can test this by comparing treated and untreated ("control") groups. However, evaluations of drug effectiveness must also take into account the "placebo effect"—whereby people feel better simply because they think they are being helped. The placebo effect can be both powerful and misleading. For example, about 30 or 40 out of every 100 people will notice an improvement in their headache even if given a sugar pill!

Confidence in a remedy can enhance its placebo effect. The patent drug industry knows this and tries hard to build up your faith in its products. Spokesmen in its ads talk like doctors. Their sales pitches use scientific-sounding words like "analgesic," "decongestant" and "anti-inflammatory agent." Whether the consumer can understand these terms doesn't matter. As long as a favorite medicine contains one or more of them—that's good enough. Many products come in fancy packages. Fancy colors, shiny capsules, special flavors, trademarks and brand names all can build confidence.

Drug-makers take advantage of people's desires to control their own destinies by "doing something" instead of letting nature run its course. Drug ads also encourage you to be your own doctor by placing labels on common symptoms. Everyone feels sluggish or tired at times. But in the hands of the ad-makers, "sluggishness" becomes a possible symptom of "kidney congestion" and "tired blood" becomes a likely cause of fatigue. It is not necessary for most people to have a bowel movement each day or on a rigid timetable. But in the hands of the ad-makers, "irregularity" becomes a symptom which needs their laxatives. People's fears of being unattractive are often aroused and exploited to sell products. Female genital deodorants, which cannot cure any underlying odor problem and are sometimes dangerous, illustrate this type of exploitation.

The use of a body part in a drug's brand name is another sales technique. Leaving the details to your imagination, such names suggest the ability to treat the body part, strengthen it, or both. *Carter's Little Liver Pills* was a classic example of a misleading brand name for the pills contained absolutely nothing that was good for your liver.

Public faith in patent medicines is enhanced by widespread beliefs that products must be effective in order to be marketed and that health advertisements must be truthful "or else they wouldn't be allowed." It is true that many blatant falsehoods have been subject to government prosecution (see Chapter 21). But the patent drug industry has generally stayed one step

23

ahead of the law. The U.S. Federal Trade Commission had to struggle for 16 years to get the word "Liver" removed from *Carter's Little Pills!*

Patent drug-makers have been remarkably effective in selling their products. One recent study reported that during a 48-hour period, 25 percent of persons in an upstate New York area had taken a non-prescription drug. Another study, done in Canada, showed that 58 percent of people questioned had used at least one non-prescription medication during the previous 48 hours. Of these, about 60 percent had taken one drug, about 25 percent had taken two, and about 20 percent had taken three or more!

Aspirin is Aspirin

Misleading sales tactics are not only used to promote products with ineffective ingredients; they are also used to sell products which contain effective ones. Aspirin is the prime example. In plain form, it is an excellent drug to combat fever and relieve aches, pains and malaise (general poor feeling). More than 100 products which contain aspirin as their principal effective ingredient are being marketed. To convince people to buy their particular product—*which invariably costs more than plain aspirin*—manufacturers add other ingredients, vary the aspirin content and make a variety of misleading suggestions.

Anacin, for example, is said to be "like a doctor's prescription" because it contains more than one ingredient. An *Anacin* tablet contains about six grains of aspirin plus the amount of caffeine found in one-quarter cup of brewed coffee. The adult dose of aspirin is ten grains. The dose for children up to ten years is one grain per year of age. Yet *Anacin* calls itself "the adult strength pain reliever."

Excedrin ads state that "in two major research studies on pain, at a major hospital and an important

24

university medical center, doctors reported that *Excedrin* worked significantly better than regular aspirin tablets." This advertisement implies that *Excedrin* is widely recognized by the medical community as being more effective than plain aspirin. The facts are otherwise:

Two *Excedrin* tablets will give you six grains of aspirin, four grains of salicylamide (which is less effective than aspirin), three grains of the aspirin substitute, acetaminophen (which is not advantageous to combine with aspirin), and the amount of caffeine found in one cup of coffee. Hardly an "extra-strength pain reliever"—as its ads also suggest. In July 1974, *The Medical Letter* (the respected publication which advises doctors) made this comment: "Combinations of aspirins with other analgesics [pain relievers], such as *Excedrin,* have never been proven more effective than the aspirin alone, and they may cause a higher incidence of adverse effects."

Buffered aspirins, such as *Bufferin* and *Ascriptin,* are supposed to prevent stomach distress by decreasing stomach acidity. But the amount of antacid they contain is quite small. A glass of water is probably just as effective as a buffer. *Bufferin's* claimed ability to dissolve twice as fast as aspirin is also of doubtful significance.

Arthritis Pain Formula and *Arthritis Strength Bufferin* contain seven and one-half grains of aspirin. This dose has no significant advantage over that of the ordinary five-grain aspirin tablet, but is more expensive.

And so on.

How Advertising Affects Pharmacists

Many pharmacists would prefer not to carry products which they feel are useless. But they feel forced to do so by consumer demand which has resulted from advertising.

Pharmacists are professionally trained in the science of drug chemistry and drug use. Their state and national organizations place great value on continuing education. Their journals contain reliable scientific information and their schools offer courses to help practitioners keep up-to-date. But pharmacists are *also* subject to the influence of advertising by patent drug manufacturers. Often these ads are profit-oriented and contain little or no scientific information. For example, one manufacturer suggests its skin creams because they are "best sellers." Another suggests stocking its antacids, laxatives and cold tablets because they are "traffic builders." Another recommends its cough medications "to get the jump on winter." Whether these products are of any value in treating the conditions for which customers use them seems not to be the point.

The typical pharmacist wears a white coat and is regarded by his customers as an authority on patent medicines. He may be very helpful when customers ask him about the large selection of patent medicines he sells. It is important to realize, however, that pharmacists do not necessarily endorse every product they sell.

The Trouble with "Tonics"

Pharmacists are not the only health professionals whose actions affect the sale of questionable patent remedies. Physicians also play a role. Many people wish that somehow a medicine could fortify them against the hardships of life. Drug advertisers exploit this hope by suggesting that their "tonics" can supply energy and fight "that tired, run-down feeling." But medical doctors also promote such concepts when they prescribe placebos for fatigue. Most of the tired feelings for which patients seek relief are caused by emotional tension. Far too often, doctors do not take the time to find out what is troubling their patients (or to refer

26

them to others who will). Instead, by using vitamins, tonics, or other substances as placebos, these doctors reinforce the myths of the tonic-makers.

The so-called "tonics" are flavored mixtures of vitamin and minerals to which proteins are sometimes added. Aside from the few calories which they may contain, there is nothing in them which can give you "extra energy." They contain no nutrients which are not readily available from a balanced variety of foods. More than one hundred of the tonics now sold, however, are not merely a waste of money; the ones which contain iron can be quite dangerous if misused.

Iron is a mineral which is needed to make hemoglobin, the substance in red blood cells which carries oxygen to your tissues. Iron deficiency anemia is found in certain segments of our population. It occurs most commonly in women who menstruate heavily, pregnant women, and people whose diets are restricted for economic or other reasons.

The only sensible reason to use an iron supplement is iron deficiency anemia. However, it is not sensible to manage this condition without medical supervision. To establish the diagnosis, a blood count is needed—and before treatment is started, it is important to look for the underlying cause. If the anemia is caused by heavy menstrual periods, the doctor might either prescribe an iron supplement or try to reduce the bleeding. If faulty diet is the problem, nutritional counseling will be in order. If the anemia is caused by internal bleeding from an ulcer or a developing cancer, however, curing the anemia without making the diagnosis might mask the more serious problem until it is too late.

Some people who use iron-containing tonics experience mild stomach irritation. But these tonics pose another more serious potential danger. Children who ingest iron tonics—thinking they are some sort of tasty drink—can undergo serious poisoning and even death.

Although it is true that iron deficiency anemia can make people tire easily, very few people who suffer from fatigue have this condition. For many years, promoters of iron-vitamin tonics have been getting away with claims that their products are appropriate for the treatment of fatigue. But in 1976, the U.S. Federal Trade Commission succeeded in having the manufacturer of *Geritol* and *FemIron* pay a high penalty for misleading advertising.

Government Pressures

Clearly, something is terribly wrong with the patent drug marketplace. Instead of educating consumers, most advertising misleads them. Many patent remedies contain no effective ingredients, many contain ineffective amounts of ingredients, and some can even be dangerous when used as directed. During the past few years, federal agencies have become increasingly concerned about this situation. As a result, scientific panels to judge the safety and effectiveness of various types of patent medicines have been appointed by the Food and Drug Administration in the United States and the Health Protection Branch in Canada.

The findings of the FDA panel on non-prescription sedative, tranquilizer and sleep-aid drugs were summarized in the December 8, 1975, *Federal Register*. North Americans have been spending more than $35 million a year for these products. The FDA study evaluated 23 of their ingredients. Vitamins and passion flower extract were noted to serve no rational purpose. Aspirin and related ingredients were judged to be ineffective for sedation. Other ingredients were judged to be unsafe because their effective dose differs little from their toxic dose. In this category were bromides (found in *Nervine* and *Alva-Tranquil*) and scopolamine (found in *Compoz, Sominex, Nite Rest, Sleep-Eze* and *Sure-Sleep*).

Certain antihistamines were recommended for further study to determine whether they can be used safely in effective dosage as non-prescription drugs. Antihistamines are used mainly to treat allergic symptoms. They can produce drowsiness as a side effect, but they can also produce constipation and dry mouth. Most people who use sleep aids do not realize that they may contain antihistamines.

The expert panel also criticized advertising for the non-prescription sedatives and recommended an end to claims that these products help such things as "nervous irritability" and "simple nervousness due to common everyday overwork and fatigue."

Seventeen expert panels have been appointed by the FDA. The sleep-aid group was the fourth to publish its findings. Its report is considered "advisory" at this point and the FDA will not issue final regulations until public and industry comments have been studied. Early in 1976, the U.S. Federal Trade Commission proposed a rule which could eventually be used to stop advertising claims which are unsupported by scientific evidence. Under this rule, claims which the FDA will not allow on labels will no longer be permitted in advertising either.

The attorneys-general of 18 states have petitioned the U.S. Federal Communications Commission to halt TV advertising of patent drugs between 6 a.m. and 9 p.m. daily. Led by Massachusetts Attorney General Francis X. Bellotti, the group charged that such advertising leads to drug abuse among children. In related testimony before the House Communications Subcommittee, Bellotti said, "Madison Avenue encourages everyone, including children, to take drugs to get up, to stay awake, to stay slim, healthy and beautiful, to eliminate minor pain or discomfort and to go to sleep."

Although these developments look promising, it is by no means certain that they will reach a successful conclusion. The patent drug industry is unlikely to give up any profitable sales tactics without a struggle.

Protecting Yourself

If you use non-prescription medicines, you owe it to yourself to do so in a scientific and responsible manner. Don't rely upon advertising claims. Before you buy a product, you should read its label and ask yourself the following questions:

1. What are its ingredients?
2. What do these ingredients do?
3. Are they safe for me?
4. Has their effectiveness been proven by scientific tests?
5. Is this product the most economical way to solve my problem?
6. Might it cause me to overlook a condition for which I should see a doctor?

If you have an illness, make sure that the patent medicine will not harm your particular condition or interact adversely with any other medication your doctor has prescribed.

Don't take patent medicines unnecessarily. Many advertisers suggest remedies for conditions which do not even exist. If patent medicines are a regular part of your life, you are probably abusing them (or vice versa). This is particularly likely if they are antacids, laxatives or tonics. Record what you learn about patent medicines in a special notebook.

Despite the questionable nature of many of its products, the patent medicine industry is booming. Its customers are spending billions of dollars a year. To keep them buying, the drug industry is spending hundreds of millions of dollars on television advertising alone. But remember, the man on the TV screen is not your doctor—or anyone else's. He doesn't know the real cause of your backache, your headache, your upset stomach or your fever. He doesn't know why you are tired. And very likely, he doesn't care.

Recommended Reading

The Medicine Show, from Consumers Union, is a practical guide to some everyday health problems and health products and contains several excellent chapters on non-prescription remedies. It is available from Pantheon Books/Random House in hardcover and paperbound editions.

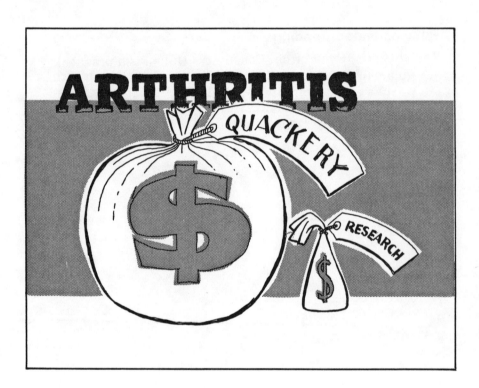

3

THE MISERY MERCHANTS

For every dollar spent on arthritis research, fifteen dollars are spent on arthritis quackery.

BY

DIANA BENZAIA
Associate Director of Public Information
The Arthritis Foundation

"Do you ache all over when you wake up in the morning? Are your joints stiff and swollen during the day? Do you fall asleep in pain? Then you don't need a doctor to tell you have arthritis. And a doctor can't cure you either. But our out-of-this-world treatment can cure you!

Government scientists have never revealed the fantastic medical benefits of soil samples brought back from the moon. But now the secret is out! This amazing moondust will cure you of arthritis—as it has cured others—and you can have it right now, without a doctor's prescription! The cure is quick and the price is cheap when you think of the happy life ahead of you—without arthritis!"

Would you believe the above sales pitch—that a single salesman has obtained closely guarded samples, that an arthritis cure is being kept secret, that a layman can cure what a doctor cannot? Let's examine it closely.

"You don't need a doctor to tell you have arthritis." False! There are nearly one hundred different kinds of rheumatic disease. Arthritis can strike at any age, even in infancy, and can last a lifetime. Proper treatment requires proper diagnosis. Symptoms similar to those of arthritis may even be caused by other types of disease. Only a qualified physician can properly diagnose and treat arthritis.

"Government scientists have never revealed the fantastic medical benefits of soil samples brought back from the moon." False! No scientist would have reason to keep an arthritis cure secret. Sharing a "secret cure" is a favorite sales trick of quack promoters.

"This amazing moondust will cure you." False! There is *no* cure for arthritis. It is common, however, for the disease to have ups and downs. Some patients, after having been troubled by pain for months, may

34

suddenly feel free of all symptoms. The absence of pain may last for days, weeks or even months. If, by pure coincidence, the patient has used a quack product just before this period of temporary improvement, he will be tempted to believe that the product has cured him.

"The cure is quick and the price is cheap." False! Arthritis victims waste more than $485 million a year on quack products. But money isn't all they have to lose. They can also lose valuable time. Although a doctor cannot promise quick results, he can plan a program of medication and physical therapy which can minimize pain, deformity and disability. Early diagnosis and treatment offer the best results. Patients who walk away from their doctor when they learn that proper treatment may be slow and limited will delay treatment that might make a crucial difference in the outcome of their disease. Those who abandon proper medical care for quackery are doomed to disappointment. Yet their chronic pain can make them desperate enough to try anything that sounds good.

Arthritis hucksters, who can do nothing but harm their victims, are truly "merchants of misery." Let's look at the various types of "treatments" they offer.

Gadgets and Devices

The supposed curative powers of various metals have been glorified by quacks for years. You may have seen arthritis sufferers sporting copper bracelets. For best results, promoters recommend wearing one on each wrist to set up a so-called "curative circuit." Pure hokum, of course, but that doesn't stop the salesman from selling or the desperate from buying.

"Magnetic induction" to cure arthritis was claimed for the "Inducto-scope." This strange device consisted of metal rings which were to be placed over afflicted parts of the body. The rings were connected by wires to

35

an electric wall outlet. The Inducto-scope had no medical benefit and also exposed its users to dangerous electric shocks. For these reasons, the U.S. Food and Drug Administration stopped its sale. The "Solarama Board" is another gadget which is based on mixed-up electronic theory. Also known as the Earth Board or Vitalator, it is supposed to be placed under the victim's mattress at night. The board supposedly emits free electrons to rejuvenate the body. Its various forms sell for $85 to $250.

Radioactive healing powers, which sound good to many laymen, were claimed by the "Vrilium tube." This was a brass tube about two inches long which contained barium chloride. It cost about a penny to manufacture, yet sold to arthritis victims for $300. The $30 "Oxydonor" claimed it could "reverse the death process into the life process" as well as cure arthritis. Buyers were told to clip metal disks to their ankles and immerse an attached cylinder in water—the colder the water the better. Victims of this fraud soon discovered that all they got for their money was cold toes.

Quacks keep up with the times by developing "new models" of their devices just as other businessmen do. The "Polorator," an electric heat-shocking machine, first appeared as a large, bulky item to be applied to areas of pain. Later it was issued as an attractive, slim metal wand with a small metal roller at one end. Needless to say, it "polarized" nothing.

Vibrators of all sorts are immensely popular with arthritis quacks. Vibrators may offer some relief of minor muscle pain caused by over-exertion or fatigue. They may have a relaxing effect on some muscular tension. But all this is just temporary. Vibrators cure nothing and can sometimes do serious harm by increasing joint inflammation. This is a far cry from the "miraculous" relief promised in some advertisements. Whirlpool baths are also sometimes promoted in misleading fashion. The moist heat of whirlpool devices may temporarily soothe aching bodies, but many which are sold are no more effective than a plain hot bath. In addition, those which fail to maintain constant temperatures may stress the patient's cardiovascular system.

Lotions, oils, creams and liniments are similarly over-rated by some promoters. These products may exert a temporary soothing effect, but advertising which suggests that they hold greater potential is a cruel deception. Such items applied to the outside of the body can have no effect upon internal body processes and therefore no impact on the course of the disease.

Diets and Food Supplements

So the food faddists try to get inside your body. There is hardly a food item which has not been promoted at one time or another as a "cure" for arthritis. Medical research has found only one form of arthritis (that of gout) which is partially related to diet. Yet myths persist that dietary factors can cause or cure other arthritic conditions.

Perhaps the most widely publicized food supplement at one point was "immune milk." This is said to get its immunity from antibodies produced by cows which have been injected with streptococcus and staphylococcus vaccines. Scientific studies have shown that this milk has no effect on arthritis, yet gullible buyers have paid up to $1.70 a quart for it. Other supplements touted for arthritis have more or less appeal, depending on your point of view. How does cod liver oil and orange juice sound? Not too good? Then the "healer" down the street will suggest honey and vinegar, or maybe molasses.

The idea of "natural" foods as beneficial to health is getting a lot of publicity these days. Diets based on raw

37

foods, foods without chemical additives and other supposedly "natural" nutrition items are being hustled by health food stores. So are misleading books which, unfortunately, have been best-sellers. "Natural" faddists overlook the fact that prehistoric man—who certainly ate no additives—also suffered from arthritis. This fact has been documented by bone studies.

So the "health" and "nature" food peddlers go on, offering alfalfa tea, sea brine, citrus concoctions, vitamin supplements and other expensive products that are absolutely useless to arthritis sufferers. In fact, promoters of nutrition nonsense sometimes harm their followers. Fad diets which omit essential nutrients or encourage avoidance of proper medical care will endanger the arthritis sufferer as they will any other person.

Folklore

Dietary myths come from our past. Before the advent of modern medicine, people looked to their environment for "cures." Knowing little about the real nature of disease, they relied on rumors of what helped their ancestors. The Indian medicine man, grandma and others may have no impact on disease. But if someone, somewhere, went into spontaneous remission while following their advice, that advice might become part of folklore. That is why some people with arthritis carry buckeyes, horse chestnuts or potatoes with them. Each is supposed to "draw out" the disease. And why others wrap themselves in the skins of snakes, wolves or wildcats.

"Burial" in horse manure is another remnant of folk medicine. Although the moist heat of manure may have a temporary soothing effect, there are certainly more pleasant ways to reach such a goal. But people don't always expect treatment to be pleasant. They may expect to suffer a bit. Maybe that's why so many submit to another old technique—rubbing turpentine over the affected areas. This also provides warmth, but offers burning pain as well, not to mention the unpleasant odor.

Of course, not all folk remedies are painful. Some of grandpa's elixirs can be quite delightful. Their high alcohol content doesn't stop pain, but may make sufferers less aware of it. But if that's your approach to dealing with pain, why not take it straight?

From Radium Mines to Real Estate Promotions

Nothing is ever "straight" about the quack's promises. Merchandisers of the "Radon-pad" claim it contains a mixture of radioactive materials from Swiss uranium mines which can reverse the arthritic process when applied to afflicted areas. It's a costly and useless device which emits less radiation than a wristwatch. Until recently ordered by the Federal Trade Commission to stop promoting radon gas as beneficial for arthritis, owners of an inactive mine in the Midwest charged outrageous prices for "treatments." Victims sat in dank caverns, supposedly soaking up helpful uranium rays. The radiation level in the mine is so low that it can have no effect on the body at all—which is fortunate—because high radiation levels can increase peoples' chances of developing cancer. Even though there is no scientific evidence that radiation helps arthritis, many arthritis sufferers traveled long distances to visit this mine.

In fact, traveling around for a cure is quite common for arthritis victims. Some seek cures from clinics and spas which offer special diets, mineral baths and even such unpleasant treatments as daily colonic enemas.

39

Some search for a climate which will ease their pain. Many patients believe the old myth that a warm climate will reduce their suffering. Real estate promoters capitalize on this belief. The fact is that there is no special climate which will help the arthritis victim.

Painkiller Promotions

In 1972, Americans spent more than $66 million for non-prescription arthritic and rheumatic pain relievers. In addition, arthritis sufferers accounted for half of the $106 million spent on plain aspirin and $411 million spent on aspirin-containing compounds. Aspirin *is* the best single medicine for people with arthritis. Taken according to a doctor's regimen, it can help reduce pain and inflammation. Simple aspirin does this all by itself—and that's all it does. Painkiller advertisements, however, often imply more. A product may be plugged as superior to its competitors because it "works twice as fast," gives "more effective relief," etc. The Federal Trade Commission has shown interest in stopping such misleading claims.

Medical Mismanagement

Some doctors harm their arthritis patients because they don't know any better, some even when they do. And in many instances, money is the root of the evil. Money is needed to train more specialists in arthritis care. At present there are only 2,000 rheumatologists in the United States, hardly enough to treat the 20 million arthritics who need their attention. So most people rely on their family doctor for arthritis treatment. Some family doctors provide good care. Others are sincere in their wish to help but are not up-to-date in their knowledge of arthritis treatment. An example of this would be a doctor who recommends removal of teeth or tonsils on the theory that they might harbor hidden infections.

(The theory that hidden tooth or tonsil infections can cause arthritis has long been disproven.)

A more common response of the untrained doctor is to sympathize with the patient, shrug his shoulders, indicate that "nothing much can be done," and recommend aspirin to alleviate pain. You can't call this approach quackery, but it often drives sufferers to quacks. People who are discouraged, and have more pain than they think they should, are often willing to try any approach which promises hope.

Shoulder-shruggers are nothing compared to the doctors who falsely promise "miracles" to arthritis victims. A prime example was Dr. Robert Liefmann, a Canadian doctor who claimed a drug he made would cure arthritis. Called Liefcort, the drug contains dangerous steroids and hormones. Most doctors know that steroids can provide arthritis patients with dramatic relief. To maintain this relief, however, it is necessary to continue and to increase the steroid dosage. Because side effects from steroids can be dangerous, and even fatal, patients who take them should be followed carefully. After paying high prices at Dr. Liefmann's Montreal clinic, patients returned home with supplies of medication to last several months—usually taken without medical supervision. As a result, many experienced infections, cataracts, adrenal shock, thinning of the bones, compression fractures, stomach ulcers, and even death. Although Dr. Liefmann is no longer living, and Liefcort sale is banned in the U.S., the drug is still being sold in Canada and Mexico.

Mexico, in particular, has many quack clinics which offer useless and potentially dangerous treatments. An estimated 120 patients a day go to the clinic of Dr. Louis Carrillo in Mexicali. Dr. Carrillo's examination usually takes only five minutes. Patients are then given prescriptions to be filled only at a nearby drugstore known as "Carrillo's." The drugs may cost several hundred dollars for a few months' supply. Dr. Carrillo tells patients they contain herbs, not steroids, but laboratory analyses prove that some do contain steroids. His patients may feel better for a while after returning home, but many develop complications such as water retention, stomach ulcers, weakening of their bones, infections and cataracts. Then they wind up in the office of an American doctor, if not a hospital or morgue, victims of arthritis quackery in its most drastic form.

Other Mexican clinics offer other dangerous drugs. Dipyrone, manufactured in Germany and sold in Mexico, is one. Dipyrone can cause agranulocytosis, a disease where the white blood count drops and infection can then lead to death. Dimethyl sulfoxide (DMSO) is another. It is an industrial solvent similar to turpentine. DMSO may provide temporary pain relief for some arthritics, but the FDA reports there is no evidence that it can benefit them in the long run. In addition, it may damage the eyes, liver, kidneys, central nervous system and other organs.

Quacks in Print

How do arthritis victims in Maine hear about clinics in Mexico? By word-of-mouth grapevine and the power of the printed word. Freedom of the press allows anyone to plug his remedy for arthritis, and quacks take full advantage of the media. Many books—including some from supposedly reputable publishers—promote false theories about the cause and treatment of arthritis. Most of them promote special diets. Authors and publishers are not the only ones who profiteer in print at the expense of arthritis victims. Newspapers and radio and television stations which accept advertisements for misleading books are equally to blame.

Acupuncture

Promotion before the facts are all in may not be as unethical as promotion of the definitely phony. But it can still be harmful. Acupuncture illustrates this. When this ancient Chinese technique arrived on the American medical scene, it was hailed as a surgical anesthetic. Then it was promoted as a cure for various ailments. Massive publicity led many arthritis hopefuls to join the long lines at acupuncture clinics, hoping for a cure. Research to date seems to indicate that acupuncture may provide temporary relief of pain for some arthritis patients—but has no long-range effect on the course of the disease. More scientific research is needed to see whether acupuncture will find a place in the list of legitimate treatments for arthritis. Until all the facts are in, many arthritis patients will be lined up for another disappointment.

Other Quasi-Medical Approaches

Irresponsible publicity has recently been given to a variety of supposed "cures" garbed in a medical aura—such as clotrimazole and vaccine therapy. The anti-fungal clotrimazole, for example, was hailed by a British physician as a cure for rheumatoid arthritis, which he said was a protozoal infection. His claims received front-page coverage in many newspapers.

Few newspapers gave much space to the follow-up, however, which revealed that: the physician involved was neither an arthritis specialist nor then licensed to practice medicine in Britain; the manufacturers of the drug he recommended reported no knowledge that it had anti-protozoal activity, even if rheumatoid arthritis were a protozoal infection, which it appears not to be; the physician had not conducted a controlled trial and did not even have any clotrimazole to dispense. Pity the poor arthritis patients who wasted thousands of dollars traveling to England for a "cure" after the first newspaper reports!

Other recent "cure" reports are also characterized by unscientific theory, lack of controlled tests and refusal to permit other physicians to examine patient records. When any such "breakthrough" is reported in the press before review by medical colleagues, the arthritis victim should be suspicious. Some "breakthroughs" may merit further investigation, but those with no scientific basis will merely raise false hopes.

The Reality of Arthritis

The arthritis victim who is disappointed by one "miracle" after another may develop a sense of hopelessness. When told that rheumatologists really *can* help him, he may react like the townspeople did to the boy who cried "wolf" once too often. He may disbelieve.

The reality of arthritis is that it is a chronic disease. When it comes, it usually stays and lasts a lifetime. It is the nation's number one crippling disease, but much of its pain and disability can be prevented through early diagnosis and proper treatment. Every patient with arthritis is different, but an individualized treatment program can be worked out for him. Most arthritis patients can be helped with a well-designed program of medication, special exercises, rest and other measures— prescribed by a well-trained physician.

What's also very real is the research now being conducted to find the causes of arthritis. To achieve this, the amount of money spent on research must be increased three or four times.

People in pain form a ready market for "miraculous" cures. For every dollar spent on research into the causes and treatment of arthritis, more than fifteen dol-

44

lars are being wasted on useless quackery. What a "miracle" it would be if this trend were reversed!

Recommended Reading

Beyond the Copper Bracelet—What You Should Know About Arthritis, by Louis A. Healey, M.D., Kenneth R. Wilske, M.D. and Bob Hansen. Published by Charles C Thomas, Springfield, Illinois. 1972. Price: $3.25.

The Truth About Arthritis Care, by John J. Calabro, M.D. and John Wykert. Published by David McKay Company, Inc., New York. 1971. Price: $6.95.

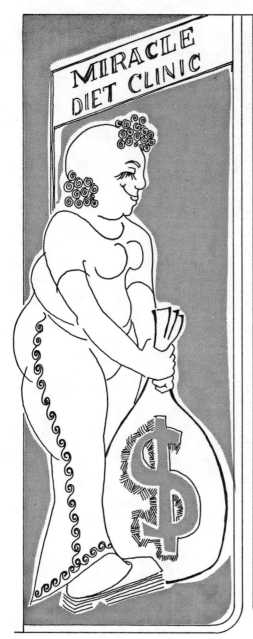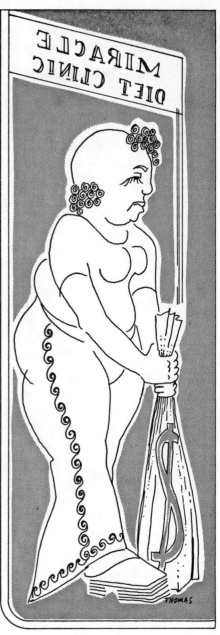

4

WEIGHT CONTROL AND "DIETS": FACTS AND FADS

Profiteers exploit the craze for thinness so that they can sell their pills, their diets and their books . . . If their miracle regimen or diet revolution entail sometimes serious risks for the consumer, what of it?

BY

JEAN MAYER, Ph.D.
President
Tufts University

Weight reduction has become a national obsession. In some ways this is quite understandable. National statistics suggest that fully half the middle-aged men and one-third their female contemporaries are significantly heavier than they were at age 25—when their growth was completed. Every pound put on since then is fat. The data specifically indicate that American women gain most weight when they are pregnant, and later, after menopause. Men gain weight gradually between 25 and 40 years of age and faster after 40. Generally this is because as one ages one needs fewer calories.

Health and insurance studies clearly show the penalties of overweight—considerably increased risk of sickness and death from diabetes, liver and kidney disease, diseases of the heart and blood vessels, and other problems. Current research indicates that the most serious problem associated with obesity is high blood pressure. However, correlations between overweight and sickness and death are not very impressive when overweight is less than 20 percent.

Children and adolescents, too, are getting fatter. In some selected suburbs of the Boston area, which we have monitored for close to 20 years, almost 20 percent of graduating seniors are overweight. While in most rural areas and in those with better all-year-round climates, overweight is less prevalent among young people, there is little doubt that the condition is on the increase. While it does not immediately carry the same health penalties during youth that it does during middle age, overweight is also a serious handicap to the young. With fashion magazines, television ads, newspaper articles and ads extolling thinness, with uniformly thin models, actors and actresses cast in romantic roles, overweight young people are made to feel unattractive and are, in fact, often rejected for positions of leadership, for dates and even, as our studies have shown, for college admission. The situation is made worse by those profiteers who reinforce and then exploit the craze for thinness so that they can sell their pills, their diets and their books. The concern of these people is not for the public health but for their own financial welfare. If their miracle regimen or diet revolution entail some (sometimes serious) risks for the consumer, what of it? They are good for the author—or his ghost writer.

Who Should Lose Weight?

This long preamble done with, let us see what can be reasonably said about weight control and diets. First, who should reduce? Just because overweight is very common and is bad for you does not mean that everybody should lose weight. Our studies in the Department of Nutrition at Harvard have taught us that a considerable number of adolescent girls and young women go on reducing diets for no good reason whatsoever. Indeed, we find that girls with large bones and muscle masses and girls with stocky builds almost invariably put themselves on diets, even when they carry no excess fat—and to an experienced observer look very good indeed. A lot of girls with builds like the younger Elizabeth Taylor or the present-day Sophia Loren feel that they must lose weight. Yet if you look like Sophia Loren, even prolonged starvation will not make you look like Twiggy or today's most popular models, and why should you want to? But the desire is there, we found, with an enormous proportion—in some samples, near totality—of normal-weight young women going on one ridiculous diet after another so that they can get into a dress one or two sizes smaller.

The genesis of this trend is clear: it has been created by dress designers and fashion magazines. An anecdote will illustrate this. A few years ago I found myself

49

at a New York luncheon next to the (female) editor of a well-known women's fashion magazine. Trying to think of subjects of mutual interest, I asked her about her models, who she informed me were on the average five feet eight and weighed 110 pounds. (The average U.S. woman who buys the clothes advertised by these models is five feet four and weighs over 125 pounds.) I asked the lady what she would do if the Venus de Milo came to the magazine looking for a job as a model. Would she hire her? "Heavens no," was the reply. "I would not even want her as a receptionist. She was much too fat." As a result of this response, during my next visit to my native city of Paris, I made a special side trip to the Louvre to take a look at the old girl. It confirmed my opinion that 2500 years after her birth, she was still as beautifully proportioned as ever. Of course, she might not be at her best in a tightly tailored suit. But in a bathing suit, an evening gown, or in her own state of *deshabillé*, she would and does look gorgeous.

There is an important moral to this. Don't diet just to please New York dress designers! Other men (fortunately, a large majority) have different appraisals of female beauty. A few years ago, in the course of a study of body image and self-image, we presented several hundred young men and as many young women with sets of male and female silhouettes, asking them to choose those they thought best. Young people of both sexes agreed on the ideal male figure. Young women, however, chose as the ideal female figure one or two "sizes" thinner than that chosen by the young men.

The net effect of an exaggerated desire for thinness (and the belief that the only way to reduce is to "diet"), is often disastrous from a nutritional viewpoint. Self-inflicted malnutrition—particularly iron-deficiency anemia—is the frequent result of an inadequate caloric

50

intake, with insufficient attention paid to those foods which provide the nutrients which young people—young women in particular—need. But more on this later.

There is an even much more acute risk to this craze for thinness. It is a condition, almost exclusively seen in young women, called "anorexia nervosa"—self-inflicted starvation which can be pursued to the point of death. The adolescent girls or young men who suffer from it are almost always bright, articulate and conscientious. They cut down on their intake (often make themselves throw up what they had eaten at the family table to please their anxious parents) and set themselves "tasks" of walking and exercising to increase further their energy expenditure. (They are bright enough to know that exercising more is as effective as cutting down on your food intake to create the caloric deficit which causes weight loss.) By the time they have lost a third of their weight, their hold on life becomes precarious. Somewhere between a 40 to 50 percent weight loss they die. Many of us think that a basic cause of this disorder is a defect in self-image, whereby they see themselves as fat. They say they are, and generally refuse to look at themselves in a mirror. When their thin arms and legs are pointed out to them, they retort by saying that it makes the rest of their body appear all the grosser. The condition is often precipitated by the thoughtless (or would-be joking) remark of a man important to them—boyfriend, father, in the case of one superb athlete I knew, her coach—that they are getting fat. Add to this a compulsive nature, which makes them stick to a reduction regimen that other girls abandon soon after they pick it up, and you have set the stage for tragedy. Less advanced forms of the condition—what the French call *formes pristes,* first sketches—are all too common nowadays.

51

Fad Diets

But let us assume that you have a weight problem, not an imaginary one but due, in truth, to more fat than you should carry for your health, comfort and beauty. What is the answer? Certainly not the succession of those faddist diets which, season after season, claim that they will enable you to lose weight and yet eat as much as you want. I constantly marvel at the gullibility of my fellow citizens for believing not only that it is possible to thus flout the laws of nature—and to do so on the basis of principles which change from year to year. I can remember diets based on the following principles:

The low protein diets: The "rice" or "Duke" diet was originally developed for the treatment of high blood pressure. It consists of white rice (boiled, unsalted) and those fruits lowest in calories. It is low in iron, contains no vitamin B_{12} or vitamin D and is a highly unsatisfactory diet in the long run. Another variant was the "Rockefeller" diet (developed at the Rockefeller Institute for an experiment; it was not meant to be a reducing diet and has been disowned by the Institute for this purpose).

The "high protein" (in fact, high fat) diet: This is a diet which comes and goes—but not, each time, without bringing notoriety and riches to somebody. It first appeared in the 1860's as the "Banting" diet and has reappeared in this era as the "DuPont" or "Pennington" diet (so named after a Doctor Pennington who used it on executives of the E. I. DuPont de Nemours Chemical Company), the "Mayo Clinic" diet (disowned by the Mayo Clinic), the "Air Force" diet (ditto for the Surgeon General of the U.S. Air Force), the Stillman "Doctor's Quick Weight Loss" diet (with eight glasses of water), the "drinking man's" diet (with martinis), and Atkins' "diet revolution" (a particularly extreme form).

52

All of these diets advocate an avoidance of foods containing starches or sugar, and claim, in effect, that protein foods, meat in particular, are essentially calorie-free or thinning. The fact is that protein, like carbohydrate, contains four calories per gram, and fat contains nine calories per gram. The calories from meat, incidentally, are derived from fat more than protein (about 75 percent calories from fat in hot dogs, 60 to 75 percent in most hamburgers, at least 50 percent in "lean" steaks). Eliminating carbohydrates causes a certain body dehydration, with rapid weight loss in the first few days due to loss of water rather than loss of "unwanted fat." (This weight, obviously, can be regained as rapidly.) Thereafter, weight loss proceeds only to the extent that you eat less than you expend—as is true in every diet. (A loss of one pound corresponds, on the average, to a cumulative deficit of 3500 calories over the course of days of dieting.) Drawbacks to this diet are: (1) The absence of carbohydrates (the nearly exclusive food of the brain) means that protein has to be made into blood sugar, a process which often leads to levels on the low side, tiredness and headache; and (2) the high saturated fat and cholesterol content of the diet is dangerous for those people who have a tendency to high blood cholesterol to start with, particularly overweight middle aged men and older women.

The "grapefruit" diet: This is "based" on the supposed ability of grapefruit, or the organic acids thereof, to eliminate the calories in the rest of the diet. While grapefruit is a good food *per se,* this theory is pure drivel!

The "hard-boiled egg" diet: You can eat all you want as long as it is a hard-boiled egg. Eggs are a good source of almost all nutrients (except vitamin C and—unless you eat the shell—calcium!). And they contain only 80 to 90 calories. After a dozen hard-boiled eggs, you

53

should be pretty sick of them—and yet you have eaten less than 1200 calories, so you should lose weight. At the same time, this variant of the high-protein, high-fat diet is extremely high in cholesterol (250 to 300 milligrams per egg) and is therefore potentially quite dangerous in the long run.

What Should You Do?

If you want to lose weight, there are five principles you should keep in mind:

First, remember that losing weight is a matter of arithmetic. Any diet (including a sane, complete, well-balanced diet) which has less calories than you expend will lead you to lose weight. A deficit of 500 calories per day will yield a weight loss of one pound a week. If you think that's not very much, remember it is 52 pounds a year—and that should be enough. Losing weight slowly means that you will not get tired in the process, stop menstruating if you are a young woman, become anemic, or generally buy a lot of trouble for yourself.

Second, remember that your diet should be balanced with enough fruits, vegetables, milk or cheese, good sources of iron, such as liver, some eggs (particularly for women) and enriched or whole grain cereals.

Third, remember that a diet is not a list of "permitted" foods which are "not-fattening." Portion size is the key. Bread is only worth 70 calories per slice. Ten slices may be too much but only one or two slices a meal would be all right. Ditto for potatoes, meat, etc.

Fourth, avoid "empty calories," those foods that contribute nothing or almost nothing to your nutrition except calories.

And, finally, remember that increasing energy expenditure is just as useful as cutting down calories—and much more fun. You can increase your energy expenditure by 200 to 300 calories per hour by walking, 400 to 700 by playing tennis or swimming. Like a bank account, what is taken out is just as important as what goes in. And it has the additional advantage of making you look taut and fit. It's much better for your health and looks to be thin and firm than simply thin and flabby. Occasional brief bouts of exercise won't do it but a well-established daily routine of walking and more active exercise several times a week is the basis of lasting fitness—and lasting looks.

Editors' Note: Resumé of Weight Reduction Methods

"Amazing diets" of one kind or another produce amazing profits for their promoters. They are all based on the fantasy that a magic combination of ingredients can cause you to lose weight no matter how much you eat. Use one and you are more likely to shed dollars than pounds.

The American Medical Association Department of Food and Nutrition lists some clues which can help you to recognize a "kooky" book or diet promotion:

1. It uses bad biochemistry.
2. It makes a heated attack on carbohydrates as bad for people.
3. It claims to be a revolutionary new idea.
4. It reports testimonials rather than documented research.
5. It refers to the author's own case histories but does not describe them in detail.
6. It claims 100% success.
7. It claims persecution by the medical profession.

Amphetamines (e.g., Dexedrine) are sometimes used to suppress appetite at the beginning of treatment. Their effect is temporary and they can have unpleasant side effects.

Artificial bulk-producing agents frequently are sold with the claim that they will curb appetite by tricking the stomach into thinking it is full. Your stomach won't be tricked, so don't you be tricked either.

Artificial sweeteners, used in place of sugar, provide another means of reducing calorie intake.

"Cellulite" spot-reduction plans are supposed to get rid of "unsightly, unevenly distributed pads and lumps of fat which dieting and exercise will not dissolve." The plans consist of diet plus exercise and massage. Exercise and the recommended diet are good for general weight-reduction, but the "cellulite" concept is mere window dressing.

Counting calories. Safe and effective, the low-calorie balanced diet is ranked highest by professional nutritionists.

Counting carbohydrates. Studies show that counting carbohydrates goes hand-in-hand with counting calories. A balanced diet that relies on lowering carbohydrate intake is fine.

Diuretics can make you lose weight by causing your body to shed water. This effect is short-lived; the weight will come back when you stop the pills. Diuretics can have bad side effects. If you want to lose fat, not water, stay away from diuretics as a "weight reducing" pill.

Exercise machines tend to be overpriced and most people find their use monotonous. Good exercise programs can help you burn up calories and improve your body tone. Passive machine exercise, however, will do little more than reduce your chances of being mugged in the park.

Formula diets (usually liquid) containing specified numbers of calories offer a simple regimen which does not require much knowledge of nutrition. They may substitute usefully for one meal a day, but most people find them too monotonous to use more often.

HCG (Human Chorionic Gonadotropin), a hormone derived from the urine of pregnant women, is neither safe nor effective. The 500-calorie diet which often accompanies injections is a semi-starvation one which is likely to result in protein loss.

Kelp, lecithin, cider vinegar and B$_6$ accompanied by a 1000-or-so calorie diet will cause weight loss—as a result of the diet alone. The kelp and other supplements are of no benefit in a weight reduction program.

Low-calorie foods can give you a bit more food with fewer calories. Non-caloric sweeteners and low-calorie dressings may make your food more interesting, but their nutritional value is negligible. People on low-calorie diets must pay close attention to the nutritive content of their foods. Choosing foods by calories alone is not a useful approach.

Obesity specialists should be approached with caution. Some are excellent, but many are overpriced and follow questionable nutritional theories. Membership in the American College of Nutrition or the American Society for Clinical Nutrition is a good sign. So is medical school affiliation. But make a fast retreat if a "specialist" suggests any of the systems criticized in this book!

Reducing clubs often offer needed moral support and nutritional information. If you join a weight-reducing club, make sure it has a consulting nutritionist.

Reducing pills (non-prescription type) imply or state outright that you can eat all you want and still lose weight. This type of false claim has made millions for some of its promoters. [Regimen tablets, claimed to shed pounds without dieting, sold for an estimated $16 million between 1956 and 1962. In the court case that ended in conviction of the manufacturer and the advertising agency, it was shown that TV models who reduced during an advertising campaign had done so by *dieting.*]

Reducing salons may give you moral support in keeping to your program of exercising, but if you can't afford one, don't use one. Exercise at home on a regular basis, but beware of over-exertion.

Sole diets—such as the fruit diet, the macrobiotic diet, or any diet restricted to one food—are unhealthy because they do not provide adequate nutrition.

Spot reducers, such as creams, sauna belts and electric shock devices, may *appear* to work by causing water loss or muscle contraction. These are temporary effects. Spot reducers do *not* roll it off, rock it off or bake it off!

Starvation diets can cause protein breakdown and are potentially dangerous.

Surgical procedures which bypass part of the small intestine are in the experimental stage. So far, the results are unsatisfactory.

Thyroid hormones in large amounts can cause you to burn calories faster, lose weight and *strain your heart.* If your thyroid is normal, small amounts of prescribed thyroid will simply cause your body to produce less of its own. Thyroid preparations must carry a label statement that they are not for use in weight reduction. If you suspect "hypothyroidism" (underactive thyroid gland) as the cause of your overweight problem (a very rare disease, by the way), have it diagnosed at once by a physician who does not rely on the basal metabolism test (BMR) to make his diagnosis.

Vitamin supplements are not necessary if you eat a balanced diet.

"Wrapping" your body so that a concentrated salt solution can take the water out of the outer layers of your skin can produce only temporary shrinkage at best. At worst, if enough of you is wrapped, you can get seriously ill from dehydration.

Your doctor may be able to help you plan a proper diet or refer you to someone else for that purpose. Registered Dietitians of the American Dietetic Association are trained in dietary counseling.

Recommended Reading

The Healthy Way to Weigh Less—a five-page pamphlet prepared by the AMA. Send 20¢ for pamphlet #OP-322 to the American Medical Association, 535 N. Dearborn Street, Chicago, Illinois 60610.

Royal Canadian Air Force Exercise Plans for Physical Fitness—Famous XBX and 5BX plans are available in one booklet. Send $1.25 to Mail Service Dept., Simon & Schuster, 1 West 39th Street, New York, N.Y. 10018.

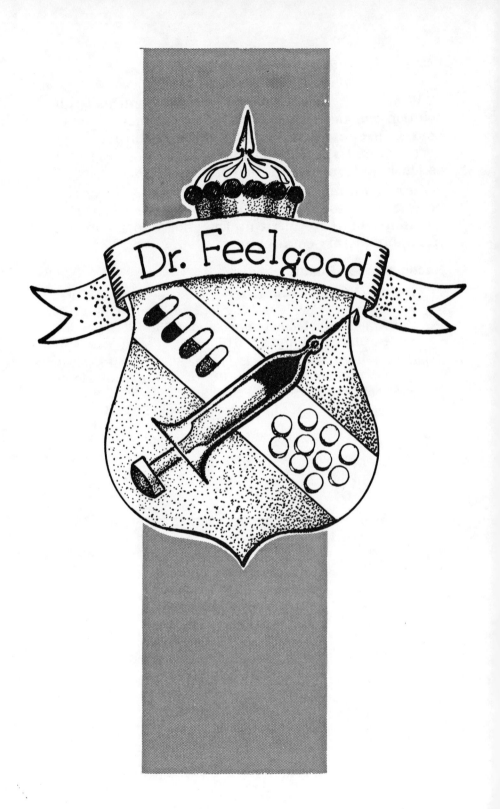

5

AVOIDING THE "MARGINAL" MEDIC

*"Quacks are the greatest liars in the world
except their patients."*
—Benjamin Franklin

BY

PHILIP R. ALPER, M.D.
Assistant Clinical Professor of Medicine
University of California Medical School

Recently a Dr. Max Jacobson lost his license to practice medicine in New York State at the age of 75. Nicknamed "Dr. Feelgood," this man had been practicing in New York City since coming to this country 30 years earlier. He was found guilty of giving injections which included significant amounts of amphetamines ("speed"). During an eight year period, Dr. Jacobson purchased a quarter of a million syringes and twice as many hypodermic needles. Dr. Jacobson often gave his shots to patients without examining them. He also took them himself. And he gave some patients drugs to take home for self-injection. One such patient, the well-known photographer Mark Shaw, died of an overdose of amphetamines.

What was striking about Dr. Feelgood's practice was that it included many of the brightest and most accomplished people of our time—"heads of nations, members of the Kennedy clan, and some of the most famous names in show business," according to a report in *Medical World News* magazine. To convince skeptics, the report included a photograph of Dr. Jacobson hiking in Florida. His companions in the picture were President John Kennedy, Kennedy's Harvard roommate Charles Spaulding, and Prince Stanislas Radziwill. The photographer had been Mark Shaw.

The Rise of Medical Standards

Fortunately, very few physicians nowadays are quacks. This wasn't always the case, however. Before 1910, there were more than 300 "medical schools" in the United States. But most were "diploma mills," from which an M.D. degree could be obtained by little more than attending a few lectures and paying a fee. Then the landmark *Flexner Report* was issued which boldly outlined the deficiencies of American medical education. The report, together with Abraham

Flexner's vigorous personal efforts for reform, resulted in the closing of 80% of the then-existent medical schools. High standards for medical training were developed and so was an accreditation system to insure that medical schools follow these standards.

Counting pre-medical education, medical training now takes from nine to fifteen years. Both the length and the intensity of this training make it very unlikely that an aspiring "quack" could complete it.

Once in practice, most physicians are subject to "peer review" by their colleagues. This process is most significant for physicians who practice in accredited hospitals. In such hospitals, "utilization" committees review the management of patients to determine if their treatment was necessary and proper. Pathologists carefully examine each bit of tissue removed during surgical operations to see if it was diseased. A practitioner who is not up to standard will hear from his colleagues and could have his hospital privileges curtailed if he does not mend his ways.

Outside of hospitals, medical societies can examine complaints—primarily involving unethical conduct—which are brought to their attention. A physician who does not adhere to the ethical standards required by his local medical society can be expelled.

Unfortunately, however, neither hospitals nor medical societies can insure that all practicing physicians are competent and ethical. For one thing, physicians tend to have a sympathy for each other which sometimes interferes with the forcefulness of self-policing. For another, it is possible for physicians to practice medicine without belonging either to a medical society or to the staff of an accredited hospital. If a doctor you consult belongs to neither, ask him to explain why. If he was expelled, watch out! If he never joined, make sure his reason makes sense to you.

63

State boards of medical licensure have the ultimate power to stop errant physicians from practicing altogether. But most state boards do not have adequate funding or tough enough laws to do this job properly (see Chapter 6).

Though I have pointed out some of the problems that the medical profession and the government have in protecting you from marginal practitioners, I would not like to leave you feeling alarmed. Very few practicing physicians are marginal and fewer yet are outright quacks.

Avoiding the Outright Quack

Long ago, Benjamin Franklin observed that "Quacks are the greatest liars in the world except their patients." Maybe that's why they are so difficult to prosecute. As I think about "Dr. Feelgood," I can't help wondering whether his patients were so ignorant or so blinded that they never suspected him. And his magic shots, available nowhere else, that made them feel just terrific—weren't they too good to be true?

Quacks are the despair of "straight" physicians. They are often charming and project a feeling of greater-than-usual concern. A charismatic quack can produce a legion of adoring clients to testify on his behalf. But certain behavior should make you suspect that a doctor has *abandoned* medical science:

—If a doctor claims to have a special machine or formula.

—If he makes blanket statements that surgery, x-rays or drugs do more harm than good.

—If he claims that other doctors are persecuting him or are afraid of his competition.

—If he advertises or uses testimonials from patients to build his practice.

64

If you encounter any of these traits, not only should you seek another doctor but you should also report your experience to your local medical society and your state board of medical licensure. What you observed may not merely be poor medical practice—it may be illegal.

The "Marginal" Medic

The above list should help steer you clear of those few doctors whose involvement with unproven methods is extreme. It is important to realize, however, that quackery is not an "all-or-none" phenomenon. A doctor who is otherwise competent may have a misguided belief in a particular medication or procedure. For this reason, it would be unwise to judge a physician's competence solely on the basis of any one action he takes.

Nor is it possible to construct a list of what would be "proper" treatment for each and every illness. Doctors are alarmed at what has been termed the "tyranny of uniform standards"—the idea of a chart or "cookbook" to follow in treating each ailment. For under such a system, physicians could not use their judgment to tailor treatment to the individual patient. Moreover, there are areas of medicine which are *genuinely* controversial.

Despite these difficulties, is it possible to detect when a doctor practices a generally sloppy or unscientific brand of medicine? Or that he is a fuzzy thinker in whose hands you would be taking an unnecessary gamble? I think so—to some extent. Your doctor's management of certain common clinical situations can tell you a lot about his thinking.

Infections And Their Management

Infections can be caused by many different kinds of germs. Some germs can be killed or weakened by antibiotics and some cannot. Generally, bacterial infections will respond to antibiotics. "Strep throat" is a

65

common example. Viral infections will usually not be susceptible to antibiotics, though there are exceptions. The common cold is an example of a viral infection which will not respond to antibiotics.

The "ideal" way to treat an infection is to identify the germ which is causing it and prescribe an antibiotic which is specific for that particular germ. A doctor can often tell which germ is infecting you by the pattern of your illness. He can be more certain of his diagnosis, however, if he takes a *culture*—whereby your germs are grown in a way that they can be positively identified. "Sensitivity" tests can then help to determine which antibiotic is likely to be most effective.

The medical school professor, speaking as a pure scientist, may want all infections cultured. But the doctor who treats many patients must be more concerned with the cost of his services, not only to individual patients but also to society's total health care budget. Where his clinical judgment can be accurate most of the time, the clinician will ask himself how much extra cost is justified for a slight increase in accuracy.

The wise physician must be prepared to use whatever tests are necessary in those conditions which require greater diagnostic precision. Bladder infections in women illustrate this point. It is usually not necessary to obtain a culture with the first such infection— particularly if the patient is a young woman who has just begun sexual activity. If the infection keeps coming back, however, cultures should be obtained to insure precise use of antibiotics. It may also be wise to obtain a kidney x-ray (known as an intravenous pyelogram) to rule out possible underlying causes of the infections.

Thus, in the overall management of infections, the important consideration may not be whether a doctor takes a culture or uses an antibiotic in a particular case. Rather, it is whether he has carefully thought out his methods of working. The wise physician will use cultures to advantage and will use antibiotics *selectively*. Complete avoidance of cultures and routine use of antibiotics for treating ordinary colds are signs of fuzzy thinking.

The Use of Tranquilizers

Articles in the medical literature point to a worrisome increase in the use of tranquilizers. Some reports, however, suggest that most patients who receive them have serious and sometimes disabling symptoms.

Many people have strong feelings on this subject. Some think it is wrong to depend upon medications. Others want quick relief. The person who simply swallows tranquilizers is missing the chance to learn about what makes him nervous and what other ways he can use to help himself. Similarly, a doctor who prescribes tranquilizers too readily—without trying to understand the nature of his patient's tensions—may be doing him a disservice.

The Use of Placebos

Placebos (sometimes referred to as "sugar pills") are substances which have no real effect on the body. Any benefits they confer are through the power of suggestion—a response to the idea that something is being done. Today it is rare for physicians to prescribe totally inactive drugs as placebos. The public is too sophisticated for this form of "psychotherapy." Instead, low doses of regular medications are likely to be used.

There are many situations where *scientific* treatment does not call for the use of medication. But some patients cannot accept such treatment. Unless they get a shot or a pill, they feel that the doctor "isn't doing anything."

Faced with such patients, ethical doctors are in a quandary. Should they give in to the patients' wishes and become unscientific physicians themselves? Or should they flatly refuse and worry that the patients will shop around until they land in the hands of a marginal or even quack physician? Either way, the doctor really can't win. It is often impossible even to debate the issues with a patient unless the doctor and patient have gotten to know one another and have developed a relationship of trust.

To illustrate the issues involved, consider the case of a married man who developed sexual impotence. This man was convinced that something serious must be wrong with his "glands." So he went to Dr. Z and pressed for a hormone shot. Dr. Z could simply have given the shot. But he did not. Instead, he performed a thorough physical examination and took a careful history.

It turned out that during a period of stress at work, the patient's potency had diminished to the point where he could barely have intercourse. Both he and his wife were modest people who found it difficult to discuss the subject of sex. The patient was ashamed of himself and afraid of "failing" again. His wife didn't want to seem forward by complaining. So they had stopped having intercourse for several months.

The physical exam revealed nothing to suggest a glandular disorder. Here, then, was a problem that was purely psychological. But when Dr. Z suggested that the patient discuss his doubts and fears with his wife, the man was crestfallen. So intense was his lack of confidence that he could barely imagine doing it. Eventually, Dr. Z and his patient struck a compromise. The doctor explained that no glandular deficiency existed, but if the patient still insisted, he would give him a hormone shot anyway. In turn, the patient promised to talk things over with his wife.

With the injection to bolster his confidence, the patient did speak with his wife. A month later, when he returned to the doctor's office, all was well. No more hormone shots were given or requested.

Some doctors might criticize the handling of this case for not being "100% scientific." But the patient was not deceived. Nor was the injection used as a substitute for confronting the real issues. *The placebo was used merely to gain the patient's cooperation.* Suppose, however, that the doctor had put the patient on a series of injections after only a brief discussion. This would have reinforced the patient's fears and probably would have made him become dependent upon medication he didn't need.

There are purists who feel that the use of *any* placebo is quackery. But the better view is to look not only at *whether* a doctor uses placebos, but *why, how* and *how often* he uses them. The doctor who uses them judiciously, but who stresses their limited value, who tries to deal with the real problems of his patients, and who tries to wean his patients, is still practicing the art of good medicine. But the doctor who gives placebos frequently when they are not requested, who makes extravagant claims for them, or who makes patients dependent upon them, should be suspect. Such practices are unethical because they *create* a demand for placebos.

Throughout this book it will be stressed that patients are usually in a poor position to judge whether a given treatment has helped them—or whether they got better with time or experienced a placebo effect. Quacks capitalize on this difficulty by crediting *all* improvement to their healing powers. Physicians rarely *try* to mislead patients in this way, but sometimes do so inadvertently. Sometimes medications are marketed which are later shown to be ineffective. But some doctors who have seen patients improve while taking these medications may mistakenly conclude that they are effective. Confidence in a drug which does not work may thus result in its unknowing use as a placebo. So there is another aspect of placebo evaluation—does the doctor who prescribes a placebo know that he is using one?

Guarding against the use of outmoded treatment is one part of what physicians accomplish by undergoing "continuing education." This means reading current journals, attending conferences and doing whatever else is necessary to keep up with medical advances. *The Medical Letter* is one publication which provides an excellent discussion of the effectiveness of treatment methods. Whether your doctor reads it is one indicator of his interest in keeping up-to-date.

Fad Diagnoses

Just as there are fad treatments, there are also fad diagnoses. A few years ago, many nervous or tired people were said to have "adrenal insufficiency"—a serious glandular disorder that is actually quite rare. Not only were the vast majority of these people misdiagnosed, but they were also treated with adrenal gland extract, a substance they didn't need and which is potentially harmful.

The search for a *magic* diagnosis goes on. Today, "hypoglycemia" (low blood sugar) is fashionable as a socially acceptable diagnosis for certain symptoms of nervousness or fatigue (see Chapter 12). "Low thyroid" is likewise unjustifiably diagnosed in many cases of fatigue. Real cases of these glandular disorders do exist, *but they are rare* and should be carefully checked by laboratory testing before the diagnosis is made. Interestingly, the few physicians who are "true believers" in these conditions simply diagnose them left and right. You should be wary of any doctor who has made any of these diagnoses on half a dozen of your friends and has them all on the same treatment. The doctor may be a poor or even unscrupulous practitioner.

Indeed, one doctor I know of, who used to diagnose adrenal insufficiency all over town, later decided the same patients had hypoglycemia. Fortunately, he is no longer in practice.

Thyroid for Weight Reduction

Thyroid hormone is sometimes used as part of a weight reduction program. Evaluation of this practice should consider why and how it is prescribed. Does the patient really have hypothyroidism as a cause of his overweight? (It is possible, but uncommon.) Is the thyroid being used as a placebo? Or is a fad diagnosis involved?

Some overweight patients insist upon "diet pills." They simply cannot accept the idea that the best way to lose weight is to develop sensible eating habits. For these patients, half a grain or one grain a day of thyroid can be used as a placebo to gain their cooperation with the rest of the weight control program. Used in this way, it is a safe and inexpensive placebo—in marked contrast to human chorionic gonadotropin injections which are commonly used at weight reduction clinics which exploit their clients.

There are a few doctors, however, who prescribe *large* doses of thyroid to patients whose thyroid function is normal. This treatment is designed to "burn off fat" by increasing your metabolism *above normal*. But this practice is dangerous because it can strain your heart and other organs. Any doctor who suggests it to you should be carefully questioned and probably dismissed.

The "Shot Doctor"

Most medications are just as effective by mouth as by injection. Shots are less comfortable and cost extra. So the *general* use of injections rather than oral medication should be questioned. Doctors who inject *most* of their patients should be suspected of poor medical practice. But note that I say *suspected* rather than *rejected out-of-hand*. For it is conceivable that some doctors who use many injections have valid reasons for using them.

The rules for judging injection use are not black-and-white. Take penicillin, for example. This drug will usually do its job quite well when taken orally, and routine use of shots will run an unnecessary risk—if the patient is allergic, a shot will produce a more trouble-some reaction. But there are times when penicillin shots are appropriate. Shots can start to work faster and may be indicated when the doctor wants the treatment to take effect as soon as possible. Shots can produce a higher blood level and are the route of choice for syphilis. Strep throats require ten days of treatment, and where patients cannot be relied upon to complete the treatment, a single shot of long-acting penicillin will do it for them.

These are just some of the many factors which a doctor should think about when using penicillin—one drug among the thousands in use today.

Complicated? Yes, it can be—but let me give you my personal guidelines for evaluating a suspected "shot doctor."

The first thing to consider is whether he is injecting medications which would be just as effective by mouth. Assuming he is, the next consideration is what stimulates the use of shots. Is it patient demand or is it his own idea? If patients demand, does the doctor resist? Some patients have such confidence in shots that refusing to give them might only result in driving them into the hands of a marginal practitioner. The better practice is to give in at first but work toward making patients less dependent upon them. If they cannot be stopped altogether, at least they can be given infrequently.

So far I am talking about effective medications. The same principles apply to placebo shots—but there is far less excuse for frequent use.

Vitamin B-12 shots are frequently used as placebos. B-12 does have a lifesaving medical use—the treatment of pernicious anemia, a *rare* disorder that affects the blood and nervous system. But other uses of B-12 are unscientific. The doctor who tells you that B-12 or "liver" shots "will really fix you up" when you feel "run down" is using them as placebos. The use of B-12 to treat iron deficiency anemia is fuzzy thinking. Surveys of doctors' practices have shown that *frequent* use of B-12 injections is often associated with poor standards of care in other areas.

I don't want to give you the impression that I am totally "against placebos." Or that you should look down on all doctors who use them. The practice of medicine is very complex and there are situations where placebos have real value. I can recall one woman whose severe problem with itching baffled both me and a topnotch skin specialist. After standard treatment failed, in desperation, we tried a B-12 shot—which worked. To this day I don't understand why. Nor do I understand why some injections (like female hormones for menopausal symptoms) sometimes seem to be more effective than the same medicine in pill form. We don't have a scientific explanation for everything we see.

The point here is that some doctors *may* have valid reasons for giving more shots than average. On the other hand, shots should not be used as a substitute for taking enough time with patients to reach an adequate understanding of their individual cases.

Sometimes I encounter people whose doctors have given them vitamin or hormone shots two or three times weekly for many months or years. Such treatment angers me. It may not be immediately clear whether such doctors are motivated more by fuzzy thinking or by greed. Either way, however, their patients have a lot to lose.

Questioning Surgery

Nowadays there is considerable discussion of "unnecessary" surgery. The most commonly questioned operations are appendectomies, tonsillectomies, hysterectomies, and procedures on the back for chronic pain. It is often pointed out that more of these operations are done in the United States than abroad. Arguments rage about whether too many operations are done here or not enough are done elsewhere. The answer is quite likely a bit of both.

In a recent New York study, an insurance company began requiring a second opinion by a specialist before it would pay for elective (non-emergency) surgery. Thirty percent fewer operations were done than before. So it is probably wise to have two opinions before agreeing to elective surgery. This does not necessarily mean that two surgeons need be consulted. A capable personal physician who is familiar with the surgeon's work will not let his patients be stampeded into an unnecessary operation. He will ask the surgeon to justify the procedure to him as well as to you.

The Skillful Patient

Licensing laws, accreditation, and peer review procedures play a major role in protecting you from marginal physicians. But no system can be perfect. To get the most out of our health care system, you must become a skillful patient. Choose your doctors with care and get into the habit of having them explain what they are doing for you—in language you can understand!

THE MAKE-BELIEVE DOCTORS

*Freddie Brant, alias Reid L. Brown, M.D., might
still be carrying on his thriving practice had he
not run afoul of the computer.*

BY

ROBERT C. DERBYSHIRE, M.D.
*Secretary-Treasurer
New Mexico Board of Medical Examiners
Past-President, Federation of State
Medical Boards of the United States*

Let me tell you a true story. Freddie Brant was born 50 years ago in Louisiana. Reared in poverty, he stopped school after the fifth grade. During World War II he was in the Army for four years. After discharge he found that jobs were scarce for a man with only a fifth grade education; so he joined the paratroops. In 1949, along with a fellow paratrooper, he was sentenced to seven years in the penitentiary for bank robbery. Working in the prison hospital, he began his "medical education." Finally released, he continued his education by working for four years as a laboratory and x-ray technician for Dr. Reid L. Brown of Chattanooga, Tennessee. There he picked up not only more medical lore but also the diplomas of his employer.

He was now ready to begin the practice of medicine. Assuming the identity of Dr. Reid L. Brown, he moved to Texas where he obtained a license by endorsement and served for three years on the staff of the State Hospital at Terrell. He then resigned and took his wife on a vacation trip. Stopping for a Coca Cola in the small village of Groveton, Texas, he treated the injured leg of a child. He found that Groveton had long been without a doctor and its people were clamoring for medical care. "Dr. Brown" soon became established as the town physician and as a community leader.

Freddie Brant, alias Reid L. Brown, M.D., might still be carrying on his thriving practice in Groveton, Texas, had he not run afoul of the computer. By coincidence he ordered drugs from the same pharmaceutical firm in Louisiana which was used by the real Dr. Reid Brown. The computer gagged when it discovered orders on the same day from physicians with identical names in Groveton and Chattanooga. Following an investigation, Freddie Brant was charged with forgery and with false testimony that he was a doctor.

The exposure of Freddie Brant caused great consternation in Groveton. But its citizens rallied around their "doctor." Many were the testimonials to his skill. According to one news report, the list of his patients included some of Groveton's leading citizens as well as farmers, loggers and welfare patients. The druggist said that many cases of hardship were caused by the arrest of Freddie. A particularly glowing testimonial came from a farmer who said, *"My wife has been sick for 14 years. We've been to doctors in Lufkin, Crockett and Trinity, and he did her more good than any of 'em. She was all drawed up, bent over, you ought to have seen her. He's brought her up and now she's milking cows and everything."*

The citizens of Groveton remained loyal to Brant. A grand jury refused to prosecute him. Authorities then brought him to trial in another county for perjury, but the case ended in a hung jury with eight members voting for acquittal. According to *Chicago's American* (7/26/68), justice was thwarted because of a "lava flow of testimonials from Groveton and Terrell to the effect that Freddie Brant was a prince of a medical man, license or no license." In an unkind cut, the same paper said that the people of Groveton should have known that Reid Brown was not a doctor because he did too many things wrong. For example, he made house calls for five dollars and charged only three dollars for an office visit. He approved of Medicare and would drive for miles to visit a patient, often without fee if the patient was poor. Besides, his handwriting was legible.

What were the secrets of Freddie Brant's success as an impersonator? They were many, but the main ones were his readiness to refer any potentially complicated case to nearby towns, a personality which inspired confidence, and a willingness to take time to listen to his patients.

Freddie Brant is only one of the many medical impostors whose records are on file at the American Medical Association library. My study of these impostors is based both upon my own experience and an analysis of the AMA's records. I have examined their backgrounds, their routes to practice, their "medical documents," how long their hoaxes were successful, how they were exposed and how the public reacted to their exposure.

Let us take a look at the typical successful impostor. His medical background might consist of a tour of duty as a medical corpsman in the Army or as a pharmacist's mate in the Navy. He might have served as a hospital orderly or as a laboratory technician. He might have obtained his medical education as a patient in a mental hospital. The sole medical background of one was service as an elevator operator in a hospital. By associating with physicians, the impostor learns enough medical jargon to fool the unwary. Our impostor must also have a good memory and a persuasive manner.

State hospitals, particularly in recent years, have provided a pathway to fraudulent medical practice. I have found six such cases. One of the most interesting is that of a man with no medical background who was hired as superintendent of a state hospital. His credentials were based solely upon a diploma stolen from a Dr. Menendez, a graduate of the University of Havana Medical School. This man might have enjoyed a long and profitable career as a hospital administrator. But he resigned after nine months and moved to another region where he obtained a position as staff psychiatrist in a state hospital mainly on the basis of his recommendations from the first state. However, his second career was cut short when his new colleagues became suspicious because of his manner and exposed him. Obviously he committed a grave error by resigning his high position as a hospital superintendent. I could not learn his reasons for doing so. Possibly he became tired of administrative duties and yearned to return to clinical psychiatry.

Whatever mild amusement I derived from the story of "Dr. Menendez" soon turned to dismay as I read on. The director of the Department of Health in the state in which Menendez was first employed, whose duty it was to pass upon the credentials of this impostor, said that the state hospital was hiring some recognized foreign doctors on a temporary basis. Obviously his examination of these credentials was entirely superficial.

While the authorities in neither state should have been taken in by "Dr. Menendez," there might be extenuating circumstances, all too familiar to members of boards of medical examiners. First, there are pressures in this country to resettle foreign physicians, particularly those who are thought to be fugitives from communism. Second, there is a universal shortage of qualified applicants for staff positions in state hospitals so that standards are lowered to permit physicians unqualified for regular licenses to fill these positions. Third, highly placed politicians often intercede for them. These three factors combine to place such pressure on boards of medical examiners that it is only remarkable that they resist as effectively as they do.

There are other reasons why state hospitals offer such good opportunities for fraudulent practice. In many states, job applicants are not required to be screened by the boards of medical examiners. Where licenses are not required, special permits to practice only in the hospitals are granted. Some states have no requirements. Where the hospital authorities are the sole judges of credentials, they have neither the facilities nor the inclination to carry out adequate investigations.

How long do impostors flourish? The files of the

79

American Medical Association contain records of at least 15 impostors who practiced successfully for over a year. There were two whose hoaxes lasted for 20 years. Perhaps the all-time champion was "Dr. J. D. Phillips" who practiced medicine in various places for 30 years. According to an article in *Coronet* (August, 1953), he fooled not only patients in 11 states, but also the United States government, several county and state health departments, and dozens of respectable physicians, nurses and administrators in various hospitals. Said *Coronet, "Rarely has a faker been unmasked more often and less permanently. Certainly no one has gone to so much trouble to remain loyal to his profession."* His medical knowledge was gained from the doctor in his home town with whom he made rounds. Said "Dr. Phillips" without undue modesty, *"So I went around with him and absorbed it all. I have a photographic memory and am not exactly dumb."*

"Dr. Phillips" served time in various penitentiaries for passing bad checks and for defrauding hotels. He used these periods to study in the prison libraries. Finally his background was so firm that he was entrusted with surgery at the Maryland State House of Correction. According to the physician in charge, he was "literally a good resident." At some time during this period he was able to steal a medical license from a physician long inactive because of illness. He then had the nerve to send an affidavit to his adopted medical school that he had lost his M.D. diploma. He was promptly sent a duplicate.

"Dr. Phillips' " downfall was finally brought about by his greed and an alert insurance agent. He was involved in an automobile accident in which he suffered injuries to his neck and arm. He was sued for $600. He countered with a $40,000 suit, demanding $35,000 to compensate him for his inability to practice medicine.

The insurance agent, disturbed by Phillips' dirty fingernails, questioned his story and he was exposed in court. His medical career is now at an end as he was sentenced to 15–20 years for perjury.

How are impostors exposed? Obviously those whose medical careers last only a few months are so inept that they give themselves away. But exposure of the experts has proven difficult and frequently happens only by accident. Several have allowed their greed to get the better of them and have tried to supplement their incomes from medical practice by various confidence games. As far as I know, Freddie Brant is the only one who has been exposed by the computer.

Surprisingly, few impostors have credentials either in the form of medical school diplomas or state medical licenses. Detailed examination of the records of 30 successful impostors revealed that only eight had bothered to steal or forge such credentials. Such oversight is amazing. I found that there is one firm in California which specializes in producing phony documents. At least one impostor was familiar with this company. He not only ordered complete medical credentials, but also turned himself into an author. He removed the pages from a book and had them rebound with his name on the cover. His fatal mistake was in failing to realize that he might be asked by a colleague to discuss its contents!

The attitude of some impostors seems to be, why bother to obtain phony diplomas when they are not necessary? I am astonished at the number of hospitals which have accepted applicants for positions without first examining their credentials. This is not confined to state hospitals. A glaring example is the case of "Dr. David William Baker" who claimed to have graduated from Temple University Medical School in 1962. From a state hospital in Idaho he went to Seattle where he worked in two hospitals for a total of three months. For two months he worked in the emergency room of one hospital. According to a Seattle newspaper, a hospital spokesman said that Baker had been hired on the recommendation of a doctor who had known him when he worked at the blood bank. The hospital only detected the impostor when it learned that the AMA had sent out a circular saying that a man named Baker was posing as a doctor. The administrator's justification: Baker claimed his credentials were in transit and he was preparing to appear before the state licensing board. Hospital officials weakly contended that Baker was not a member of the staff but worked in the emergency room where he was always under the supervision of another physician.

As I studied case histories, I was struck by how many people were gullible enough to lend money to impostors. I was astonished by the readiness of bankers, whom I had always regarded as paragons of caution, to help impostors start their medical practices. In one instance a physician was the victim when he lent an impostor a considerable sum. Also fair game are citizens of many small towns with desperate shortages of doctors who will lionize any presentable individual who claims to be a physician.

Once he has begun to practice, of course, the impostor relies on the fact that most patients who do not look seriously ill will recover by themselves. This enables him to fool many people into thinking that he has given them treatment. If he is friendly, if he shows interest and compassion, and if he quickly refers to specialists those patients who do seem quite ill, the impostor is likely to develop a loyal patient following. In fact, many people will come to "swear by him." So much so that even when he is exposed as a fraud, they will defend him and be grievously hurt because the authorities have removed their "trusted family physician."

Typical is the case of the fraud who, for some six years, successfully practiced in a small town in New York State. His following of devoted patients was large. He even won the esteem of his colleagues who frequently called upon him for consultations. When he was finally exposed by the agents of the State Board of Medical Examiners, the anguished cries of his devoted followers could be heard all the way across the Hudson River. They even circulated petitions to prevent him from being banished. Nevertheless he was brought to justice and convicted of fraud.

The reactions of these people and of those in Groveton, Texas, to the unmasking of Freddie Brant are by no means isolated examples. Such reactions are particularly prevalent in small towns. One can only speculate as to why these victims of hoaxes adopt such defensive attitudes. Possibly they feel they must justify their faith in the impostor to avoid the appearance of stupidity in the eyes of their neighbors. Possibly, they are like the victims of other confidence games who refuse to report the operator because of their own personal embarrassment. Or possibly, they may genuinely feel they have been helped.

Another difficulty in exposing medical impostors stems from the indifference of the district attorneys. Apparently these law enforcers are not enthusiastic about pursuing people whom they regard as petty criminals, and this is how impostors are regarded in many states. Only in Florida, Kentucky, New Mexico and Rhode Island is the practice of medicine without a license defined as a felony. In the other 46 states it is a misdemeanor. I remember one instance in which my board of medical examiners discovered a man who was practicing without a license. On two different occasions the investigator for the board obtained receipted bills, copies of prescriptions, and samples of drugs the man had been dispensing, certainly more than sufficient evidence for the conviction of this fraud. But the district attorney showed no interest in prosecuting him. It was not until some two years later, *after the impostor had been responsible for the death of a patient,* that the state police arrested him on a charge of manslaughter for which he was convicted and sentenced to five years in prison.

The attitude of newspapers towards some impostors is interesting. While they make every effort to report the facts accurately, their stories sometimes contain a strong underlying note of amusement. In the case just cited, after the impostor had been arrested and charged with manslaughter, the local paper printed a feature in its Sunday edition based upon an interview in the jail cell of the felon. This took the form of a human interest story which depicted the impostor as an amusing eccentric and all but ignored the charge of manslaughter.

Up to a point, many of the tales of impersonation *are* amusing, provided the reader is not one of the authorities who has been duped. But the time must come when one has to be serious, particularly when one thinks of the dangers that impostors pose to the public. Freddie Brant, alias "Dr. Brown," tried to justify his conduct by saying, *"I never lost a patient."* Didn't he? How can he know? Another famous impostor, M. L. Langford of Jasper, Missouri, pointed out in his defense that he performed no surgery and referred any patient who might have complications. But could he always recognize complications or foresee them? Impostors *do* kill people, albeit not always as dramatically as the notorious Dr. Frank who was implicated in five deaths in Chicago. He was a former mental patient who persuaded a physician to help him obtain a listing with a medical referring service. He then took over the practice of a vacationing doctor. (See the *Chicago Tribune*, 12/3/58.)

A natural question is, what motivates these people to impersonate doctors? The immediate answer of the cynic is that they do it to make money. While it is true that some yearn for the imagined rich and easy life of the doctor, this is not the only answer. Some envy the authority and social position of the doctor. Others are mentally deranged, many having served terms in mental hospitals. Freddie Brant simply said, *"I always wanted to be a doctor."*

Up to this point, I have confined myself to the methods used by medical impostors. Let us now look at how they can be controlled. Obviously, as in disease, the best cure is prevention. Today several agencies are responsible for proper screening of physicians. The most important of these are the state boards of medical examiners, the medical societies and the hospitals. It should be primarily the duty of the medical boards to see that all who seek to practice medicine in their states are qualified. More careful screening of applicants for positions in state hospitals should be carried out, preferably by the licensing boards. The boards must make sure that all applicants have genuine credentials. Documents must not be accepted on faith. No matter how convincing the applicant appears to be, his documents must be investigated at their sources. The investigations should be systematic, beginning with insistence upon completion of a detailed application blank which must include a notarized statement from the applicant that he is indeed the person whose credentials he is presenting. It is important that the physician be required to present at least two photographs, one to be affixed to the application, the other to be filed for future reference in case of a question of identity. As an added precaution, the board might insist that the photograph be affixed to the application form before it is returned to the medical school for certification or, in the case of licensure by endorsement, to the board issuing the original license. Thus his photograph can be compared with photos filed previously.

Another important method of preventing licensure of impostors is the use of the personal interview. In states which license large numbers of physicians it might be difficult for the administrative officer to interview all of them. In these states the interviews could be divided up among the members of the board. Although opinions differ about the value of the interview, an experienced person should be able to learn much by observing a candidate. He can train himself to recognize certain danger signals such as poor personal grooming, vague answers to specific questions concerning medical subjects, and failure to identify properly professors in the school from which the applicant claims to have graduated.

Still another method of detecting impostors is the requirement that all applicants for licensure be fingerprinted. At present, only seven medical boards require this. Many boards feel that the professional man should not be embarrassed by such an indignity. But this is not as drastic a requirement as many think and most applicants submit to it with good grace. After all, fingerprinting is required in applications for many jobs, particularly those associated with the federal government. Robert Sprecher, writing about licensure problems in the legal profession (*Federal Bulletin,* Volume 55, pages 188–200, 1968), made an interesting observation. The mere requirement that applicants be fingerprinted will encourage them to admit to previous conviction of crimes. For example, bar examinations were given in Michigan and Illinois at the same time.

Michigan had 281 applicants, Illinois, 273. Both states asked applicants whether they had ever been charged with a crime or arrested. In Michigan, where finger-printing is required, 28 people (10%) admitted to previous arrests or convictions. In Illinois, which did not require fingerprinting, only two (less than 1%) made such admissions.

If the practice of medicine without a license were a felony instead of a misdemeanor, as it is in most states, some impostors might be deterred.

Finally, how can impostors be detected after they have established their practices as physicians? Until recently, the most authoritative source of information about physicians has been the Department of Investigation of the American Medical Association. Its files kept complete biographical records of all physicians from the time they first entered medical school until they died. If they dropped out of medical school, this was also noted. After graduation, up-to-date records were kept of internships, residencies, types and places of practice, and of any difficulties physicians might have had with the law, their boards of medical examiners and medical societies. Records of graduates of foreign medical schools who came to this country were also kept. Furthermore, at the request of a hospital, medical board or medical society, the Department of Investigation was able to conduct a complete search to determine whether or not a person was really a physician. A typical investigation involved reference to the active file, the new name file, the AMA directory, and the medical student drop-out file, in addition to a meticulous examination of at least nine other directories. If the suspect's name could not be found by such an exhaustive investigation, one could be certain he was not a doctor. Many an impostor was brought to light by such a search.

On May 1, 1975, as an economy measure, the AMA abolished its Department of Investigation and dispersed its functions among other departments. In view of the Investigation Department's many years of excellent service, I have misgivings about its fragmentation. Will this prove to be false economy?

Though medical impostors are rare, and some regard them with amusement, we must not forget that they are potential killers. Medical examining boards, hospital staffs and medical societies must take every precaution to keep their number to a minimum.

PHONY SEX CLINICS

The main stimulant to sexual quackery seems to be money. Whenever you have thousands of people who are willing to spend money, begging somebody to take it, somebody will always oblige—at a minimum of $25 an hour. Thus, sexual quackery. The current field of sexual therapy is dominated by an astounding assortment of incompetents, cultists, mystics, well-meaning dabblers, and outright charlatans.

BY

WILLIAM H. MASTERS, M.D.
Director,
Reproductive Biology Research Foundation

I had a nightmare several years ago. It was while my associate, Virginia Johnson, and I were preparing our second book, *Human Sexual Inadequacy.* That book described more than 11 years of clinical experience with couples who had visited us at the Reproductive Biology Research Foundation, in St. Louis, Missouri, seeking help in solving various kinds of sexual problems. Before we began our work it was rare that any physician would offer to treat sexual problems in the direct, specific, intensive way that we developed; and in my nightmare I saw this new branch of medicine growing suddenly into a major public fascination.

I saw it becoming a subject of television interviews and cocktail-party conversations. I saw hordes of prospective patients going to their doctors and asking, "Where can we get this kind of treatment? Is there a clinic nearby?" And I saw the doctors sadly shaking their heads: "Sorry. The field is still too new. There aren't enough trained people yet. . . ."

Warnings were issued that a deluge of patients might be forthcoming: patients demanding a type of help which would not be readily available unless the medical profession had been adequately prepared to give it. The point was made that a fourth of American medical schools failed to include, in their curricula, even a cursory discussion of sexual functions. It was urged that training of competent professionals begin right away.

Not many took the warning seriously—back then. Today, everything feared has come true. In fact, the situation is even worse than we expected. The deluge of patients has materialized, and the medical profession hasn't been able to handle it. What wasn't predicted is the enormous size and sustained insistence of the public demand for sexual therapy. The would-be patients, frustrated in their search for legitimate treatment, understandably haven't been willing to wait until it becomes available. They have gone in search of paradise wherever it was promised, looking for a happiness and satisfaction bound to sexual fulfillment. But, too often, instead of the garden of earthly delights they envisioned, they have found only their own private nightmares.

The main stimulant to sexual quackery seems to be money. Whenever you have thousands of people who are willing to spend money, begging somebody to take it, somebody will always oblige—at a minimum of $25 an hour. Thus, sexual quackery. The current field of sexual therapy is dominated by an astounding assortment of incompetents, cultists, mystics, well-meaning dabblers, and outright charlatans.

In the less than five years since *Inadequacy* was published, approximately 3,500 to 5,000 new "clinics" and "treatment centers" devoted to sex problems have been established in the United States. Of these, the most charitable estimate cites perhaps 100 that are legitimate. Our instinct says that 50 would be a better guess. Only 50 out of a possible 5,000 offer treatment methods that have been developed with proper scientific care; have been subjected to long, conscientious testing and evaluation; and are administered by trained, fully competent personnel.

The rest of the clinics offer little more than a superficial sex education at best and dangerous quackery at worst. They offer unevaluated theories, mystical cant, pop-psychology remedies, and simplistic pseudoscience. Although some of the untested approaches sound imaginative, appealing, and interesting, and some of the practitioners can present seductively logical-sounding justifications for their theories, few or none can offer a truly believable promise that they will lighten your sexual difficulties. They can promise only to lighten your wallet.

Let me support these pessimistic remarks with another set of statistics. *Inadequacy* reported that 48 percent of the patients seen in the prior decade-plus had experienced failure in previous therapy. In the past two years, among new patients visiting the foundation, the record of prior therapeutic failure has risen to 85 percent.

What do these figures tell us? Either that many more people are visiting therapists than had been previously, or that more of the therapists are inept—or both. We suspect that both are true.

Many men and women in both the medical and legal professions share our pessimistic view of the current sex-therapy scene. Among them are Louis Lefkowitz and Stephen Mindell, attorney and assistant attorney general, respectively, of New York State. A little less than two years ago, they conducted an undercover investigation of what they called "unregulated therapists"; public hearings followed.

"We have found," said Mindell, "what appears to be a shockingly widespread pattern of 'sex therapy' wherein male therapists encourage female clients . . . to engage in sexual activities with them, under the guise that this is necessary for the client's well-being." Lefkowitz reported that the roster of self-styled therapists in his state included "criminals and mentally ill persons" as well as unqualified practitioners.

A physician came to the hearing and told of a therapist who induced a woman to engage in mutual masturbation with him, because this would cure her "mistrust" of men. A college professor reported that at one institution men and women gathered in encounter groups and screamed "Hate, hate, hate!" at each other. The institution not only accepted patients for a fee, said the professor, but also offered to train apprentice therapists and to give them diplomas and degrees—

although the school wasn't accredited by the state. An undercover investigator for the state reported on a group-therapy "community" in which the patients "are urged and advised by therapists to . . . leave their homes and move in with others in the group."

Some clinics advertise or privately assure prospective patients that their therapists have been trained at the St. Louis foundation. The phrase, "Masters-and-Johnson-trained therapists" often crops up in promotional material. In most cases, this is a patent falsehood. The foundation's training methods are necessarily time-consuming. It takes anywhere from four months to a year or more to complete a course of training, depending on the man's or woman's previous clinical experience. To date, we have only eight therapy teams that have been trained in St. Louis and are practicing elsewhere in the country. When a nonauthorized clinic uses the "M-J-trained" gimmick, the phrase often means only that somebody there has read one of the foundation's textbooks.

Other therapy shops advertise that they offer treatment based on "the M-J-technique." This, too, is usually less than true. There isn't really any such thing as "the M-J technique." We follow no formula in St. Louis. We preach no dogma. We certainly aren't wedded to any therapeutic fad such as nude group-encounters or punching people to relieve anger. We treat each couple as a unique relationship, and we don't know what approach will be followed until we know what the particular problems are.

When somebody tries to hook patients with "M-J technique" as the bait, he may mean merely that his approach bears some outward procedural similarity. The foundation accepts only couples for treatment, not individual men or women. The relationship, rather than the separate individuals, is treated. Each couple stays at a local hotel and daily visits the foundation for two weeks of intensive treatment, after which comes five years of follow-up—for a total cost of $2,500 per couple. A minimum of 20 percent are treated at reduced fee or at no cost.

You may wonder why there is such concern about the sorry state of this field. What harm do sex charlatans render, after all? It isn't as though they endanger people's lives or even, in most cases, people's physical health. Although the Lefkowitz-Mindell investigation turned up some cases of severe mental disturbance and even suicide as apparent results of bad therapy, such cases are relatively rare. On the surface, it may seem that sexual quackery is fairly benign: that it takes people's money but in other respects is usually harmless.

Not so. Sex-therapy quacks can make it more difficult for legitimate therapists to help a person. Having once been in the hands of an incompetent therapist, a patient may experience special difficulties in any later treatment. For instance, the foundation staff has seen many couples who claim that either one or both partners had been seduced by self-licensed therapists. Some of these seductions have been homosexual. One troubled woman told us that a female "therapist" had induced her to cooperate in a series of sexual acts, under the pretext: "Maybe your trouble is that you're a latent homosexual. Let's check it out." Having lived through this, the woman was frightened of what might be done to her in St. Louis.

An obverse kind of problem also can arise. Instead of being frightened as a result of past encounters, some people seem disappointed to learn that seduction isn't a part of our approach. Whether apprehensive or dissatisfied, such patients represent frustrating difficulties for us. Time must be spent undoing the results of past blundering.

Another kind of problem, less measurable but perhaps even more serious, arises from the delicate, intensely personal nature of sex therapy. It takes courage to go through such therapy. If the initial experience is bad—if it yields unsatisfactory results or, worse, is actually frightening or depressing—that man and woman may never again seek help. They are doomed to live the rest of their lives with a sexual problem that might have been handled quite quickly and easily if they had only sought legitimate help from the beginning.

There is no way to measure this kind of damage. We can't count the numbers of people who, after disappointments and scares, thenceforth shy away from what could be genuine help. There are no statistics to offer. We can say only that the problem exists and that it is widespread and serious.

You ask: All right, why not drive all these frauds and blunderers out of the field? Why not sue them, prosecute them, expose them by name?

We have now arrived at the very heart of the problem. Legal action is next to impossible because there is no legal definition of what is and isn't a legitimate sex therapist.

No state, to my knowledge, has any law requiring that a self-styled sex therapist be licensed, that he conform to any minimum standards of education or experience, or that he observe any special code of professional ethics. The states license and regulate various professional titles such as "psychiatrist" or "psychologist." If you go into practice and call yourself a psychiatrist, you must be one and prove it. But should you call yourself a "sex therapist" or "psychotherapist" you can operate in most states with no restrictions beyond those that would apply to a candy-store proprietor or any other business person. As long as you behave yourself, pay your taxes, don't perpetrate provable fraud, and avoid the trap of practicing medicine without a license—avoid prescribing medicines, for example, or giving advice about a patient's kidney functions—then you can probably count on a peaceful and profitable career.

This lack of standards, this absence of either government controls or professional self-regulatory mechanisms, was the focal point of the Lefkowitz-Mindell investigation in New York. The attorney general sadly pointed out that in his state, as in most others, there is no way to protect the public from therapeutic quacks as long as they are careful. "They are within the law," he said. "Or more accurately—the nonlaw."

The main purpose of the New York hearings was to determine, in effect, whether the fields of sex counseling and general psychotherapy could or should be more strictly regulated. Some witnesses said yes and some said no, and of those who said yes, no two agreed on exactly how the purpose might be accomplished. Thus things remain at a standstill not only in New York but nearly everywhere else. Mrs. Johnson and I feel a direct and heavy responsibility for this new field of medicine, but, to date, have been frustrated in almost all attempts to protect it. Casting about for legal weapons with which to attack charlatans, we find our corner virtually empty.

Unless and until your state protects the field with a strong wall of law, there is only one man or woman who can effectively guard you against sexual quackery: That is yourself. The best advice is that, before signing up for any course of sexual therapy, you seek counsel from four separate sources:

96

Your physician. At the outset, he is probably the man best qualified to help you judge what your personal needs are. From talking to patients and other local physicians, he also may know of a nearby clinic that he can recommend.

Your city or county medical society. This organization will probably be able to recommend a clinic or at least some sources of further advice. Also, in its position as a local medical-listening-post, the society will know of at least some charlatans in the area and can help you avoid them.

Your local family and children's service. This is the focal point of social work in the area and serves as a listening post much like the medical society. Its workers will have dealt with troubled people who have had both good and bad experiences with sex therapists.

Your minister, priest, or rabbi. As a counselor to the troubled, he is likely to have helped other people grapple with marital and sexual problems, some perhaps similar to yours. He may know which local treatment centers produce results and which don't.

Even with these four sources to guide you, however, you still will need to tread warily. But we are optimistic enough to think that this will not always be the case. Back in 1910, most branches of medicine were in about the same state as sexual therapy is now. There was a chaotic lack of standards. It took a lot of time and a lot of struggle, but today most branches are fairly firmly regulated by both law and self-imposed ethics. You are reasonably safe in assuming that a man who calls himself "M.D." really is one, and that the degree means he went through a specified amount of training. The same is true of specialist titles such as "gynecologist" or "ophthalmologist." One day, perhaps, it will also be true of "sex therapist."

97

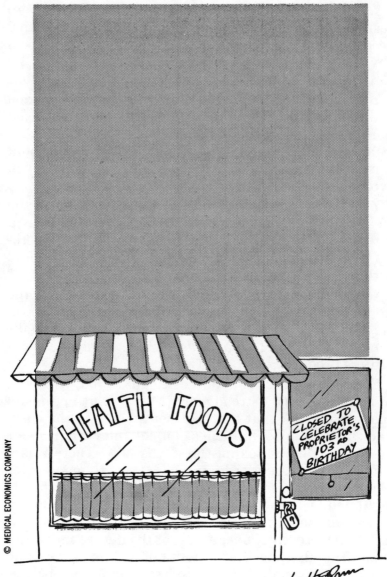

© MEDICAL ECONOMICS COMPANY

8

THE HEALTH HUSTLERS

Did you ever stop to think that your corner grocery, fruit market, meat market and supermarket are also health food stores? They are—and they charge less for food which is identical or superior to that provided by "health food" stores!

BY

VICTOR HERBERT, M.D., J.D.
*Clinical Professor of Medicine and
Clinical Professor of Pathology
Columbia College of Physicians and Surgeons*

We are being had. Most of what we read and hear about nutrition is wrong. Yet nutrition sells more magazines than sex!

We are in the midst of a vitamin craze. The health hustlers are cleaning up by stoking our fears and stroking our hopes. With their deceptive credentials, they dominate air waves and publications. The media hosts love them. Their false promises of super-health draw audiences of millions.

The situation now appears even worse than it was a decade ago, when the U.S. Food and Drug Administration Commissioner, George P. Larrick, stated:

> "The most widespread and expensive type of quackery in the United States today is the promotion of vitamin products, special dietary foods, and food supplements. Millions of consumers are being misled concerning the need for such products. Complicating this problem is a vast and growing 'folklore' or 'mythology' of nutrition which is being built up by pseudo-scientific literature in books, pamphlets and periodicals. As a result, millions of people are attempting self-medication for imaginary and real illnesses with a multitude of more or less irrational food items. Food quackery today can only be compared to the patent medicine craze which reached its height in the last century."

"Health food" rackets cost Americans over a billion dollars a year. The main victims of this waste are the elderly, the pregnant, the sick and the poor.

The "Basic Four" of Good Nutrition

Have you been brainwashed by the hucksters? Do you supplement your diet with extra nutrients? Why?

100

Do you believe that, "If some is good, more may be better"? Do you believe, "It can't hurt"? Do you believe you are getting "nutritional insurance"? If you believe any of these things, you have been brainwashed.

The fundamentals of good nutrition are simple: To get the amounts and kinds of nutrients to maintain a positive state of health, all you need to eat is a moderate amount of food from each of the four basic categories (the "four basics"). Your daily average should be:

1. Fruits and/or vegetables and/or fresh fruit juices: four or more servings.

2. Grains and/or grain products (including cereals, breads, rice, macaroni, etc.): four or more servings.

3. Meats and/or meat products (including fish and/or poultry and/or eggs): two or more servings.

4. Milk and/or milk products: Two to 4 servings. (Except for infants, the requirement for this group is now recognized as more modest than previously believed.)

An easy way to remember the four basic categories is to think of a cheeseburger with lettuce and tomato—it has them all.

The health huckster doesn't tell you that the normal person needs no vitamin supplements if he gets the "four basics" each day. Why? Because his profits come from withholding that truth. Unlike your family doctor, he does not make his living by keeping you healthy, but rather by tempting you with rash, extravagant and false claims. Such claims raise his personal appearance fees and sell the products of companies in which (unknown to you) he may have a financial interest.

The Dangers of Excess Vitamins

When on the defensive, the quack is quick to demand, "How do you know it doesn't help?" The reply to this is "How do you know it doesn't *harm*?" Many substances which are harmless in small or moderate doses can be harmful either in large doses or by gradual build-up over many years. Just because a substance (such as a vitamin) is found naturally in food does not mean it is harmless in large doses. In fact, an entire book has been written on this subject (*Toxicants Occurring Naturally in Foods, 2nd Edition,* published by a subcommittee of the National Research Council, National Academy of Sciences).

What do scientists mean by "excess" vitamins? They are referring to dosage in excess of the "Recommended Dietary Allowances (RDA)" set by the Food and Nutrition Board of the National Research Council, National Academy of Sciences. The Recommended Dietary Allowances are the "levels of intake of essential nutrients considered, in the judgment of the Food and Nutrition Board on the basis of available scientific knowledge, to be adequate to meet the known nutritional needs of practically all healthy persons."

RDA's should not be confused with "requirements." They are actually more than most people require.

Quacks charge that the RDA's are set by a group which has a "conflict of interest to work to benefit the food industry." If you ever hear this, don't believe it. The RDA Committee of the Food and Nutrition Board consists of recognized nutrition experts from the Universities of California, Iowa, Wisconsin, New York State and Harvard as well as from the National Institutes of Health and the U.S. Department of Agriculture. There is not one representative of industry on the RDA Committee. Its work is supported by the National Institutes of Health, but members themselves serve without pay. Meeting at regular intervals, the RDA Committee sets its values after thorough study of the best evidence that scientists all over the world have developed. The only legitimate use of vitamins in excess of the RDA's is in treatment of medically diagnosed vitamin deficiency states—conditions which are rare except among the poor, especially among those who are pregnant or elderly.

Too much vitamin A can cause lack of appetite, retarded growth in children, drying and cracking of the skin, enlarged liver and spleen, increased intracranial pressure, loss of hair, migratory joint pains, menstrual difficulty, bone pain, irritability and headache.

Prolonged excessive intake of vitamin D can cause loss of appetite, nausea, weakness, weight loss, polyuria, constipation, vague aches, stiffness, kidney stones, calcifying of tissues, high blood pressure, acidosis and kidney failure which can lead to death.

Large doses of nicotinic acid or nicotinamide, recommended by purveyors of "orthomolecular psychiatry" can cause severe flushing, itching, liver damage, skin disorders, gout, ulcers and blood sugar disorders.

Excess vitamin E can cause headaches, nausea, tiredness, giddiness, inflammation of the mouth, chapped lips, GI disturbances, muscle weakness, low blood sugar, increased bleeding tendency and degenerative changes. By antagonizing the action of vitamin A, large doses of vitamin E can also cause blurred vision. Vitamin E can also reduce sexual organ function—just the opposite of the false claim that the vitamin heightens sexual potency. (This claim is based on experiments with rats. . . Quacks don't know that what may be true with rats may be just the opposite with man!)

Another way to look for health trouble is with large doses of ascorbic acid—vitamin C. Here the quacks take great pleasure in attempting to link themselves with one of the truly great men of our age, Dr. Linus Pauling, two-time Nobel Prize winner. Pauling's belief that vitamin C has value against the common cold has some validity, but its value is quite limited. Like an antihistamine tablet, in some cases it may reduce the symptomatology of a full-blown cold or completely eliminate the symptomatology of a mild cold (thereby creating the impression that no cold occurred). There is no reliable evidence that large doses of vitamin C *prevent* colds, and it is therefore not logical to take such doses in the absence of a cold.

Our laboratory has just published evidence that large doses of vitamin C can destroy substantial amounts of vitamin B_{12} in food. If enough of your B_{12} is destroyed, you may develop a *very* dangerous deficiency. In addition, excess vitamin C may damage growing bone, produce diarrhea, produce "rebound scurvy" in newborn infants whose mothers took such dosage, produce adverse effects in pregnancy, and cause kidney problems and false positive urine tests for sugar in diabetics. There may be other adverse effects. What should you do? Don't take more than 45 milligrams (mg) of ascorbic acid a day (the adult RDA) unless you have checked with your doctor, are pregnant (RDA 60 mg/day) or are breast-feeding (RDA 80 mg/day).

Health Hustlers are Usually Charlatans and Quacks

The Random House Unabridged Dictionary of the English Language says that a charlatan is "one who pretends to more knowledge or skill than he possesses; quack." It then defines a quack as "1. a fraudulent or ignorant pretender to medical skill. 2. a person who pretends, professionally or publicly, to skill, knowledge, or qualification which he does not possess; a charlatan. 3. being a quack: a quack psychologist who complicates everyone's problems. 4. presented falsely as having curative powers: quack medicine. 5. to advertise or sell with fraudulent claims."

The quack's pretense to greater knowledge or skill than he really has comes in various forms, some quite subtle. For example, the pretense often comes in the form of impressive-sounding credentials. It is typical for the talk show host to remark, when a quack and a genuine scientist are brought together as guests, "You both have such excellent credentials, and yet you make diametrically opposed statements. What is the layman to think?" What the layman should think is that one of the "experts" is very likely a quack.

Often the talk show quack will support his case by quoting the findings of a "great scientist" (another quack) who has "published over a hundred studies in scientific journals on vitamin E (or whatever)." Be cautious. He may be referring to publications which will publish anything submitted by almost anybody. Many journals do not have review systems to screen out garbage. The scientist knows which journals are scientific and which ones are not. The layman may not know this. But the quack does not care about the quality of his sources of information. He merely accepts any findings which appear to support him and rejects any evidence which contradicts his ideas.

Some quacks have a more modest-seeming approach, "I have published a few papers on this—maybe it takes more papers to convince some people." Don't let this fool you. It is not the number of papers which determines scientific truth, but the quality of the contents of each paper. One thousand poorly designed studies are one thousand pieces of junk. One well-designed study is worth its weight in gold. (The quack hates well-designed "controlled" studies.) Also keep in mind that when a quack refers to his own "research," what he really means is his unscientific combination of thoughts, plagiarized from two or more sources.

Recognizing the Quack—Fourteen Tips

How can you spot the health hustlers, the food quacks, the con men, the charlatans? The following should make you suspicious:

Tip #1: He advises that you go out and buy something which you would not otherwise have bought.

Ask yourself whether the friendly fellow with the benign smile who is recommending large doses of vitamin C or E, or some other vitamin or combination of vitamins, might have a financial interest in a vitamin company or two. Next time you hear someone on a talk show pushing a vitamin, call or write the station and ask whether he or the station has a financial interest, direct or indirect, in one or more companies selling vitamins. You might also ask whether Old Toothy Smile has ever been convicted of practicing medicine without a license. And whether any company in which he has or has had a financial interest has ever had its vitamin products seized by the FDA for mislabeling. The silence which greets your inquiry will astound you.

Tip #2: He is a Fake Specialist, with Imposing "Front" Titles. Credentials sell people. Because he knows this, and sometimes because he has grandiose character traits with messianic feelings, the quack often provides himself with impressive-sounding titles. Such include "Director" or "President" of the "X Nutrition Institute" or the "Y Nutrition Society," or "Nutrition Consultant" or "Nutrition Expert" or "World's Foremost (or Greatest or Leading) Nutritionist." Be suspicious of such titles. The "Institute" or "Society" will usually prove to be a "front" (created by the quack or his agents) with no standing among genuine nutrition scientists. The titles and institutes are rarely affiliated with legitimate scientific or academic institutions. When the quack is a "Nutrition Consultant," it

106

will usually turn out to be to an organization which peddles misleading health information and/or vitamins and/or health foods. Often, the organization is controlled by him.

Information on who incorporated an institute or society is available from the State Attorney General where the institute is located. As for the title, "World's Foremost (or Greatest or Leading) Nutritionist," there is no such title given by any reputable scientific organization. It is a "cover" anyone can use, no matter how ignorant he may be about nutrition. There is no law against it, just as there is no law against anyone calling himself "World's Foremost Lover."

Some reputable organizations which work for the advancement of science will accept any private citizen as a member. Quacks often join such groups in order to add "legitimate" credentials to their list. In order to protect the public, "open" membership organizations should forbid advertising of membership. The American Association for the Advancement of Science is one which does this. Anyone who publicizes AAAS membership is likely to receive the following letter from its business manager:

> "It has come to my attention that you list yourself as a member of the American Association for the Advancement of Science in certain printed matter. It is my duty to bring to your attention the fact that several years ago, our Board of Directors passed a resolution forbidding members to advertise the fact of their membership.
>
> The reason for this resolution was that this Association will accept anyone's application for membership and, therefore, membership in this Association does not indicate any scientific

achievement of the individual. On the other hand, the reader of the printed matter, not knowing the Association's non-existing membership requirements, most likely will misinterpret the announced membership of an individual in this Association as an indication of his scientific status.

Please remove at once all printed matter which lists you as a member of our Association from circulation and prevent reference to your membership in this Association in any public statements. Thank you in advance for your cooperation."

The largest private (non-government) group of genuine health research scientists in the world is probably the Federation of American Societies for Experimental Biology (FASEB). The American Institute of Nutrition (AIN) is the nutrition branch of FASEB, and the American Society for Clinical Nutrition (ASCN) is the clinical nutrition arm of AIN. These three organizations screen out quacks, so be suspicious if a "nutrition expert" does not list one of them among his credentials—especially if he includes some other group with "Nutrition" in its title. Some quacks try to seem more respectable by attacking other quacks.

Your doctor may be able to help you separate good nutrition information from nutrition nonsense. Unfortunately, a doctorate degree is not a guarantee of reliability. A few people with M.D., D.D.S., or Ph.D. after their names—who have received their training in reputable institutions—have strayed from scientific thought. Some of them have written books. The medical and dental degrees of Emanuel Cheraskin and the dental degree of W. M. Ringsdorf, Jr., did not prevent them from writing *New Hope for Incurable Diseases,* a book which stimulates false hopes that vitamins can cure various diseases which, at present, are incurable. An advertisement for this book deceptively states that, "In an era of increasing faddism and misinformation about foods, the reader will benefit from the authoritative treatment of the subject contained herein." Unfortunately, the law does not protect you from this type of deception. When this ad was sent to the New York State Attorney General and the FDA, both replied that it was out of their jurisdiction. In the Fall, 1972 issue of the *Journal of Nutrition Education,* Dr. C. E. Butterworth, Jr., Director of the Nutrition Program at the University of Alabama (where Cheraskin and Ringsdorf are on the dental faculty), wrote a devastating review of their book, closing with:

> "There are a number of other statements throughout the book which are patently erroneous or misleading . . . The main objection to this book is the tone and attitude of the presentation. There are subtleties and innuendoes readily apparent to an educated reader but which, alas, are likely to be missed by the lay public. One expects more from university professors who write interpretations of science for the general public. This book has apparently been written for the faddist fringe and "health" food store market and for readers who seemingly *want* to believe the miracles wrought by diet without regard for scientific evidence.
>
> Surely hope is an essential element of life, both to the sufferer from an incurable disease and the members of his family. But it is cruel to raise false hope under any pretense. In my opinion, this book raises nothing but false hopes, many of them not even new, in the mind of an unedu-

cated reader. This can be grasped only by reading the entire book. I recommend this as an
exercise . . . for critical readers having knowledge of nutrition in the hope that it will stimulate them to take measures to combat misinformation. It is not recommended for the
general public to whom it is directed."

*Tip #3: He says that most disease is due to a bad or
faulty diet.* This is not so. Inspect any medical school
textbook of medicine or ask your doctor. They will tell
you that most diseases have nothing to do with diet.
Malaise (feeling poorly), tiredness, lack of pep, aches
(including headaches) or pains, insomnia and similar
complaints are usually the body's reaction to emotional
stress, overwork, etc. The persistence of such complaints is a signal to see a doctor to be evaluated for
possible underlying physical illness. It is not a signal to
add vitamins.

*Tip #4: He says that most people are poorly
nourished (the old "Sub-Clinical Deficiency" gambit).*
This is an appeal to fear which is not only untrue, but
ignores the fact that the main forms of "poor" nourishment in the United States are undernourishment in the
poverty-stricken and over-nourishment in the economi-
cally well-to-do. The poverty-stricken can ill afford to
waste money on unnecessary vitamins. Their food
money should be spent on the "basic four" which contain not only all the vitamins in proper amounts, but also
the other necessary nutrients.

It has been alleged that our advertising age has produced an addiction to snack foods, making a well-
rounded diet exceptional rather than usual. This is an
exaggeration, since the "basic four" need not be obtained in each meal, but rather over the course of an
entire day. It is true that some snack foods are mainly

110

"empty calories" (sugar without other nutrients). But it should be noted that acquiring the "basic four" is not all that difficult.

There is one form of poor nourishment which is particularly common in this country—fluoride deficiency. Fluoride is necessary to build strong teeth which resist decay. The best way for people to get an adequate amount of this essential nutrient is to adjust community water supplies so that the fluoride concentration is about one part fluoride for every million parts of water. Strangely, the quack is usually opposed to water fluoridation (see Chapter 11). It almost seems as if when he can't personally profit from the sale, he isn't interested in your health.

The quack tells you that everyone is in danger of "subclinical deficiency." Does that sound scary? It is meant to be. It is a typical sales tactic, like that of the door-to-door furnace huckster who tells you your perfectly good furnace is in danger of blowing up and you can only be saved by replacing it with his product. Scientists sometimes use the term subclinical deficiency to refer to the situation of a patient on the road to deficiency from an inadequate diet. But no normal person eating a well-balanced diet each day is in any danger of "subclinical vitamin deficiency." As one well-controlled study reported, vitamin B complex and liver supplements "produced no improvement of . . . well-being and no decline in the incidence of minor illnesses among apparently healthy people on an adequate diet."

Tip #5: He tells you that soil depletion and the use of chemical fertilizers cause malnutrition. If a nutrient is missing from the soil, a plant just does not grow. Chemical fertilizers counteract the effects of soil depletion. The quack is dead wrong when he claims otherwise! He is also wrong when he claims that plants grown with natural (animal) fertilizers are nutritionally superior to

111

those grown with synthetic fertilizers. The only "extra" you may get from an animal fertilizer is a good case of salmonella diarrhea or gastrointestinal parasites. Moreover, "natural" foods are more likely to have molds growing on them which produce aflatoxins which are among the most potent carcinogens (cancer-producers). Some food additives reduce the growth of these molds.

Don't make the mistake of thinking that the law forces people to tell the truth about nutrition. FDA regulations forbid only *labeling* claims that a deficient diet may be due to the soil in which a food is grown. But our laws do not protect you from the quack who states the same thing on TV or radio or in a publication.

Tip #6: He alleges that modern processing methods and storage remove all nutritive value from our food. This is a gross distortion of fact. It is true that food processing can change the nutrient content of foods. But the changes are not so drastic as the quack, who wants you to buy his supplements, wants you to believe. While some processing methods destroy nutrients, others add them. As long as you select your foods properly, you will get all the nourishment you need.

The quack distorts and oversimplifies. When he tells you that milling removes B vitamins and iron, he does not bother to tell you that enrichment puts them back. When he tells you that cooking destroys nutrients, he does not tell you that only a few nutrients are sensitive to heat. Nor does he tell you that these few nutrients are easily obtained by having fresh fruit, vegetable or fruit juice each day.

Tip #7: He says that you are in danger of being poisoned by food additives and preservatives. This is a scare tactic designed to undermine your confidence in food scientists and in government protection agencies. The quack wants you to think that he is out to protect you. He hopes that if you trust him, you will buy what he

112

recommends. The fact is that the tiny amounts of preservatives used to protect our food pose no threat to human health.

This chapter cannot cover this subject in detail, but I would like to comment on how ridiculous quacks can get about food additives, especially those which are found naturally in food anyway. Calcium propionate, which is used to preserve bread, occurs naturally in Swiss cheese. The quack who would steer you toward (higher-priced) bread made without preservatives is careful not to tell you that one ounce of Swiss cheese, which you may eat in a sandwich, contains enough calcium propionate to retard spoilage of two loaves of bread. Similarly, the organic food quack who warns against monosodium glutamate (MSG), does not tell you that wheat germ is a major natural source of this substance.

Tip #8: He tells you that if you eat badly, you'll be OK if you take a vitamin or vitamin and mineral supplement. This is the "Nutrition Insurance Gambit." It is dangerous nonsense. Not only is it untrue, but it encourages careless eating habits. The cure for eating badly is a well-balanced diet. Money spent for a vitamin or mineral supplement would be better spent for a daily portion of fresh fruit or vegetable. With one exception, the "four basics" diet contains all the nutrients, known and unknown, that normal people need. (The exception involves the mineral iron. The average American diet contains barely enough iron to meet the needs of infants, women of child-bearing age and, especially, pregnant women. This problem can be solved simply by cooking in an iron pot or eating iron-rich foods such as soy beans, spinach, liver and veal muscle.)

Tip #9: He recommends that everybody take vitamins or health foods or both. The nutrition quack belittles normal foods. He does not tell you that he earns his living from such recommendations—via public appearance fees, endorsements, sale of publications or financial interests in vitamin companies, health food stores and/or "organic" farms. On the subject of "health food" stores—the term itself is deceptive. Did you ever stop to think that your corner grocery, fruit market, meat market and supermarket are also health food stores? They are—and they charge less for food which is identical or superior to that provided by "health food" stores!

The quack often makes nutritional claims for bioflavinoids, rutin, inositol and other such food extracts. These "non-essential" ingredients have no recognized nutritional value, and the FDA forbids nutritional claims for them in labeling.

Tip #10: He claims that "natural" vitamins are better than "synthetic" ones. This claim is a flat lie and anyone who makes it should be immediately classified by you as a quack. Each vitamin is a chain of atoms strung together as a molecule. Molecules made in the "factories" of nature are identical to those made in the factories of chemical companies.

Tip #11: He promises quick, dramatic, miraculous cures. The promises are usually implied or subtle—so he can deny making them when the Feds close in. Such promises are the health hustler's most immoral practice. He does not see, know, or want to know the people who have been broken financially or in spirit—by the elation over his claims of quick cure followed by the depression when the claims prove false. Nor does the health hustler keep count of how many people he lures away from proper medical care.

Quacks will tell you that "megavitamins" (huge doses of vitamins) can cure many different ailments, particularly emotional ones. But they won't tell you that the "evidence" supporting such claims is unreli-

114

able because it is based on inadequate investigations and other forms of sloppy research.

Tip #12: He uses testimonials and "case histories" to support his claims. We all tend to believe what others tell us about their personal experiences. When you hear someone claim that product X has cured his cancer, arthritis or whatever, be skeptical. He may not have actually had the condition he names. If he did have the condition he names, his recovery most likely would have occurred without the help of product X. (Most conditions recover with just the passage of time.) Establishing medical truths requires careful and repeated investigation—with well-designed experiments, not reports of what people *imagine* might have taken place. That is why testimonial evidence is forbidden in scientific articles.

Symptoms which are psychosomatic in origin are often relieved by any product which is taken with the suggestion that it will relieve the problem. Most headaches and minor aches and pains will respond to any enthusiastically recommended nostrum. For these problems, even physicians may prescribe a placebo. A placebo is a substance which has no pharmacological effect on a normal person, but is given merely to satisfy a patient who supposes it to be a medicine. Sugar tablets and vitamins (such as B_{12}) are commonly used in this way.

Placebos act by suggestion. Unfortunately, some physicians, like most laymen, really "believe in vitamins" beyond those supplied by a good diet. Those who share such false beliefs do so because they confuse placebo action with cause and effect.

Talk show hosts give quacks a tremendous boost when they ask them, "What do all the vitamins you take do for you personally?" Then, millions of viewers are treated to the quack's talk of improved health, vigor

115

and vitality—with the implicit point: "It did this for me. It will do the same for you." A most revealing testimonial experience was described during a major network show recently which hosted several of the world's most prominent promoters of nutritional faddism. While the host was boasting about how his new eating program had cured his "hypoglycemia," he mentioned in passing that he no longer was drinking "20 to 30 cups of coffee a day." Neither the host nor any of his "experts" had the good sense to tell their audience how dangerous it can be to drink so much coffee. Nor did any of them suggest that some of the host's original symptoms might have been caused by caffeine intoxication.

Tip #13: He espouses the "Conspiracy Theory" and its twin, the "Controversy Claim." The quack claims he is being persecuted by orthodox medicine and that his work is being suppressed. He claims that orthodox medicine or the AMA is against him because his cures can cut into the incomes doctors make by keeping people sick. Don't fall for such nonsense. There is so much more medical business available than we doctors can handle that we import from other countries about as many doctors each year as we graduate from our own medical schools. Moreover, many doctors in health plans receive the same salary whether or not the patients in the plans are sick—so keeping their patients healthy reduces their workload but *not* their incomes.

The quack claims there is a "controversy" about facts between himself and "the bureaucrats," organized medicine and/or "the establishment." He clamors for medical investigation of "his" claims (ignoring the negative results of all past investigations). In reality, there is no fact controversy. The collision is between his misleading statements and the facts. The gambit, "Do you believe in vitamins?" is one way in which he tries to increase confusion. Everyone "believes in vitamins."

The real question should be "Do you need additional vitamins beyond those in a well-balanced diet?" The answer is no.

Any physician who found a vitamin or other preparation which could cure sterility, heart disease, arthritis, cancer and the like, could make an enormous fortune from such a discovery. Not only would patients flock to him, but his colleagues would shower him with prizes and awards—not the least of which would be the tax-free $100,000+ Nobel Prize!

Tip#14: He is legally belligerent. The majority of "nutrition experts" who appear on TV talk shows and whose publications dominate the "health" sections in bookstores and health food stores are quacks and charlatans. Why are they not labeled as such? Ralph Lee Smith, a former investigative reporter who became Associate Professor of Communications at Howard University, answered this question in the December 16, 1965 issue of *The National Reporter*. Writing in *The Vitamin Healers,* a hard-hitting article which ripped the lid off Carlton Fredericks, Smith said it is the "question of libel":

> "A reputation for being legally belligerent can sometimes go far to insulate one from critical publicity. And if an attack does appear in print, a threat of libel action will sometimes bring a full retraction. Carlton Fredericks frequently threatens to take libel action against those who disagree with him. So assiduous has he been in this respect that he even writes threatening letters to physicians who have questioned his ideas in private correspondence."

If a "nutritionist" travels with a lawyer and threatens libel actions against those who disagree with him, he is probably a quack.

As Smith noted, the threat of a libel action can be particularly effective when made against scientific and scholarly publications, especially those which are sponsored by publicly supported societies and universities.

Dena C. Cederquist is Chairman of the Department of Foods and Nutrition at Michigan State University. In March 1964, she testified at the hearings on health frauds and quackery held by a U.S. Senate subcommittee: "My salary is paid by the State of Michigan to teach, and yet on advice of our lawyer at the University, I did not write a criticism of the book *Calories Don't Count* [by Dr. Herman Taller who was subsequently convicted of mail fraud, conspiracy and violating FDA regulations] for he said I would be liable and we simply could not afford this kind of thing." She further stated about a paper relating to food faddism, presented by Kennth L. Milstead of the FDA to the American Dietetic Association in October 1962, that, "He submitted this paper first to the Journal of the American Dietetic Association and secondly to the Journal of the American Medical Association, and both organizations refused to publish it, a paper full of facts. They refused to publish it for fear of being hauled into court in one of those long, drawn-out law suits . . . , and so this very valuable bit of information which should have gone to all practicing dietitians in the United States—and could well have been read by all physicians, was not made available for publication."

The public feels that doctors should speak out against nutrition quacks because they have "nothing to fear" from a libel suit from a quack. Nothing to fear? Successful defense against a libel suit can take three years and cost the doctor $10,000 or more. We need "Good Samaritan" laws to cover the cost of defending libel actions brought by quacks! We also need vigorous enforcement of the laws against malicious prosecution. Any physician or genuine nutritionist who is sued by a quack should consider a counter-suit for malicious harassment.

This writer was threatened in connection with the 1974 David Susskind TV show "The Vitamin Craze." Just before the show was taped, I was handed a nutrition book written by a velvet-suited, silky-voiced co-panelist whom I had never heard of before—one Gary Null. After perusing it, I stated, "This book is garbage." Null immediately threatened me with a lawsuit if I repeated the statement. He told me he travels with two lawyers just to take care of people like me. Calling one of them over, he introduced us and asked his lawyer to watch me closely and hit me with a lawsuit if I said anything "out of line." Null told me he was "Director of the Nutrition Institute of America" and had 36 Nobel Prize winners on his board of directors. I replied that his Institute sounded like a quack "front" and that I did not believe it had 36 Nobel prize winners on its board. (Subsequent investigation proved that I was correct on both counts.) With this warm-up, we went on the air. It was a lively program—one of the few in which the public heard immediate rebuttal of nutritional misinformation.

The Weakness of the Law

Anybody can state, in any medium of his choice, any false, misleading or deceptive health information he chooses. The First Amendment (freedom of speech) protects him against the consequences of the harm he does, unless the false information is on the label of a product or the fraud occurs in the course of a provable doctor-patient relationship. Thus, the U.S. Food and Drug Administration, which can act against misleading labels, has no jurisdiction over misleading books.

Can the Federal Communications Commission (FCC) or the Federal Trade Commission (FTC) attack nutrition misinformation via laws which require broadcast-ers to operate in the public interest as well as laws which require "truth in advertising"? The FCC usually acts only after receiving complaints, and *a public that does not know it is being misinformed cannot complain*. The FTC appears to act only against very gross forms of advertising deception or deceptive trade practice. It does not appear to act against subtle forms of misleading information, and many complaints it receives are shelved for "lack of agency manpower." Purveying deceptive misinformation for profit appears on its face to be a deceptive trade practice. The FTC should be able to move against those who profit from public appearances in which they purvey false, deceptive or misleading nutrition information.

Why do the State Attorneys General not act? Isn't the presentation of misleading nutrition information perpetrating a fraud on the consuming public? If the First Amendment does not protect smut speech and writings which are alleged to injure mental health, why does it protect misleading nutrition speech and writings which can be proved to be harmful to both mental and physical health? When quack books were brought to the attention of the New York State Attorney General, however, he merely referred them to the FDA (which, of course, did not have jurisdiction over them).

The FDA has pointed out that excess vitamins can hurt you. How many Americans know this? How many preachers of nutrition gospel have ever mentioned this on a television talk show? This failure to mention should be prosecuted as negligence chargeable not only to the huckster, but also to his talk show host and sponsoring network. It also seems possible that the States and/or their courts can revise or interpret their "reckless endangerment" statutes to include reckless endangerment of public health by promotion of dangerous nutritional ideas. I also wonder whether the more

120

dangerous of the quack's misrepresentations could be enjoined as a public nuisance. Perhaps a public-spirited prosecutor will try these approaches someday.

Under our civil laws, it may be possible for a private citizen to recover substantial damages if he relied on misinformation purveyed by the quack to the detriment of his health. He would need to establish that the quack had a duty not to mislead him. If a doctor recommends a remedy, he has a duty both to use care in selecting it and to warn of complications. If a patient is harmed because his doctor fails to do either one of these, he can sue for malpractice. Is it too much to expect that the unlicensed quack can be held responsible for the harm *he* does?

A recent California case has created a precedent which can be cited by anyone who has been harmed by following the advice of a nutrition quack when given in a broadcast. In *Weirum* vs. *RKO General, Inc.*, the Supreme Court of California upheld a jury verdict of $300,000 against a radio station. The station had offered a cash prize to the first person who could locate a traveling disc jockey. Two teenagers spotted the disc jockey and tried to follow him to a contest stopping point. During the pursuit, one of the cars was forced off the road, killing its driver. The jury found that the broadcast had created a foreseeable risk to motorists because its contest conditions could stimulate accidents. Many radio and television stations which broadcast nutrition quackery have been put on notice by scientists that they are creating an unreasonable risk of harm. Such stations might have serious difficulty defending themselves against suits by injured listeners.

When the charming quack does have an interest in a vitamin company, you can be sure that the labeling of his products makes none of the health benefit claims which he makes on the air or in his publications. This is because our laws forbid nutritional misinformation or outright lies only in connection with the sale of products. One way to find out whether someone on the air or in a book is telling the truth is to send him a label from a bottle of a vitamin preparation he sells. Attach the label to a sheet of paper stating the claims he makes for the product (in positive terms, such as "This preparation will cure the following illnesses _ _ _ ."). Ask him to sign the statement and return it to you with the label still attached. If he does not do so, you may assume that he is afraid that his signature on *labeling* can get him prosecuted for false statements.

Quacks project an aura of sincerity and public interest. They spout (unprovable) "case histories" and tales of personal experience. They cite sloppy research as "the great work of great men." Yet their deceptions dominate the media.

The food quack benefits only himself, collecting large fees for his public appearances, publications or "consultant" status to health food and vitamin companies which he often controls. The public is not only milked financially (for more than a billion dollars a year), but may also suffer damage from vitamin overdosage and from seduction away from proper medical care.

There is nutritional deficiency in this country, but it is found primarily among the poor, particularly among those who are elderly, are pregnant or are small children. These groups need to have their diets improved. Their problems will not be solved by the panaceas of the huckster, but by better nutritional practices. The best way to buy vitamins and minerals is in the rational combination packages provided by nature: the "basic four" of (1) fresh fruits and vegetables; (2) meats, fish and fowl; (3) whole grain or enriched bread and cereal; and (4) milk products. A cheeseburger with lettuce and tomato contains the basic four.

Contrary to the health hustler's claim that "It may help," his advice not only does not help, but may harm—both your health and your pocketbook. He will continue to "rip off" the American public, however, until the communications industries develop sufficient concern for the public interest to expose his quackery. And if the media cannot develop adequate social conscience on their own, they should be forced to do so by stronger laws and more vigorous law enforcement.

Recommended Reading

The Great Vitamin Hoax, by Daniel Tatkon.

The Nuts Among the Berries, by Ron Deutsch (A history of food quackery).

Nutrition for Today, by R. Alfin-Slater and L. Aftergood.

The Bellybook, by James Trager.

Eating for Good Health, by Fredrick J. Stare, M.D.

The Family Guide to Better Food and Better Health, by Ron Deutsch.

Let's Talk About Food, by Philip L. White.

Megavitamin and Orthomolecular Therapy in Psychiatry, Task Force report of the American Psychiatric Association. ($3.00 from Publications Services Division, APA, 1700 N. 18th Street, N.W., Washington, D.C. 20009.)

Recommended Dietary Allowances, National Academy of Sciences. ($2.50 from Publishing Office, National Academy of Sciences, 2101 Constitution Avenue, Washington, D.C. 20418).

List of Nutrition Books, Recommended, Recommended for Special Purposes, Not Recommended. Reliable guide to nutrition books. Compiled by Chicago Nutrition Association. ($2.00 from Chicago Nutrition Association, 8158 South Kedzie Avenue, Chicago, Illinois 60652).

Nutrition Misinformation and Food Faddism. A collection of 17 papers published by the Nutrition Foundation. ($2.50 from Nutrition Foundation, Office of Education, 888 17th Street, N.W., Washington, D.C. 20006).

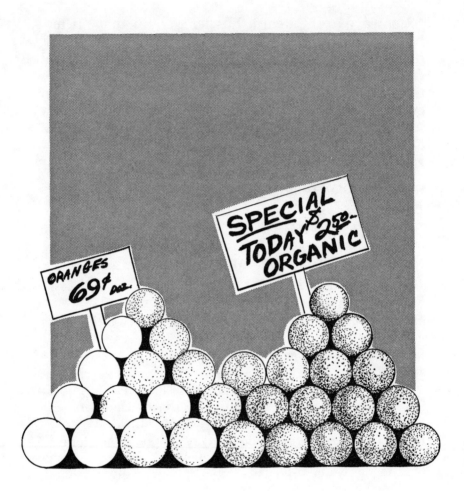

9

THE GENUINE FAKE

Pollution remains the Number One issue in the mind of the public . . . Business is beginning to see profit in supplying more natural products . . . we can exert a pincer effect—the fear of pollution on the one side and the promise of profit on the other.

— Robert Rodale
Prevention Magazine, 1971

There has not been one case of illness in America which can be attributed to a scientific agricultural procedure. In contrast, in countries where "organic" fertilizers (such as human waste) are used, food poisoning from disease organisms is quite common.

BY

THOMAS H. JUKES, Ph.D.
Professor of Medical Physics
University of California at Berkeley
and
STEPHEN BARRETT, M.D.
Chairman, Board of Directors
Lehigh Valley Committee Against Health Fraud, Inc.

In these days of high prices, you certainly don't want to waste money when you shop for food. Foods labeled "organic" or "organically grown" usually cost more than "regular" foods. Sometimes they cost twice as much—or more.

Are they worth their extra cost?

One way to begin our inquiry would be to ask what the "organic" labels mean. Unfortunately, it turns out, there are no exact industry standards. Even promoters of the organic food industry are aware of this problem. In December 1972, New York State Attorney General Louis Lefkowitz held a public hearing on the matter of organic foods. Robert Rodale, one of the nation's foremost organic and health food promoters, testified as follows:

> *"When the organic idea boomed in popularity several years ago . . . we became aware that misuse of the word organic was becoming a problem. We knew that some dealers in health foods were using the word without any intention of having it mean that foods so labeled were produced without the use of synthetic fertilizers or poisonous pesticides . . ."*

After describing how Rodale Press executives arrived at the definition which they now promote, Rodale presented the following:

> *"Organically-grown food is food grown without pesticides; grown without artificial fertilizers; grown in soil whose humus content is increased by the additions of organic matter; grown in soil whose mineral content is increased by the applications of natural mineral fertilizers; has not been treated with preservatives, hormones, antibiotics, etc."*

Let's look closely at the components of this definition to see if they make sense.

126

"Without Pesticides"

This part of the definition relates to the fear that many people have that pesticides may threaten their health. Organic promoters *imply* two things: (1) that the use of pesticides is bad and dangerous; and (2) that foods grown under "organic" conditions will contain no pesticides.

The Rodale Press definition does not actually state that organically-grown foods are *free* of pesticides. But it is clear that many retail sellers of the products make that claim. Vincent White, Confidential Investigator for the New York State Bureau of Consumer Frauds and Protection, spoke on this point at the Lefkowitz hearing:

> Q. *Mr. White . . . in the course of your official duties, did you make a survey of health food stores selling organic food in and around the area of New York City?*
> A. *Yes sir.*
> Q. *. . . visiting approximately 25 stores . . . in the guise of a customer who is interested in learning why you should purchase organic food?*
> A. *That's correct, sir. . .*
> Q. *Did you find a pattern of representation existed . . . as to the virtues of organic food?*
> A. *Yes, sir, the general consensus was that they were pesticide free . . .*

Dr. Elmer George, Director of the New York State Food Laboratory, was also a witness at the hearing. Dr. George reported that 17 out of 55 (30%) "organically" labeled products purchased at health food stores by government agents contained pesticide residues. This contrasted with an average pesticide incidence of only 20% in foods tested in his laboratory which had not been labeled organic.

Leaders of the organic food industry know that their products contain pesticide residues. When questioned, they will admit this, as did Rodale Press nutritionist, Dr. Mark Schwartz:

> Q. *You are going on the assumption . . . that there are no chemicals in organic foods?*
> A. *It is almost impossible to come up with foods that do not contain pesticides.*

Thus, if you buy "organic" labeled foods in the hope of avoiding pesticides, you are likely to be unsuccessful. But don't let this trouble you. Government agencies keep watch on our food supplies to be sure they are safe to eat. The pesticide content of today's food is not a threat to our health. The amounts of pesticides found in our foods are *extremely* small. They would not even be detectable if it were not for the exquisite sensitivity of modern measuring equipment which can measure some substances in parts per *trillion!* Moreover, it is clear that pesticides have a greater margin of safety than many other substances found naturally in foods which you and I eat all the time without worrying about them.

"Without Artificial Fertilizers"

Organic promoters suggest that natural fertilizers are better able to nourish plants and that they produce more nutritious foods. They also suggest that natural fertilizers contain, or might contain, some ingredient found in nature but lacking in artificial fertilizers. These ideas are good sales gimmicks, but nothing more. The exclusion of "artificial" fertilizers and the inclusion of "natural" fertilizers has no logical basis. From the plant's point of view, it makes no difference where its food comes from. Chemicals are taken up and used by the plant only in their inorganic chemical state no matter whether they are fed to the plant in manure, compost or manufactured fertilizer. All the plant cares about is whether it has enough food to grow. If it does, it will grow. If it does not, it will not grow.

Experiments conducted at the Michigan Experiment Station for ten years, at the U.S. Plant, Soil and Nutrition Laboratory at Cornell University for 25 years, and at the British Experimental Farm for 34 years, all indicate that there are no differences in major nutrient content whether foods are grown on soils fed with animal or synthetic plant foods. The amount of vitamin C in apples, for example, cannot be made equal to that of oranges by the addition of any amount of fertilizer. This is because nutritional factors (other than minerals) are controlled by genes (the plant's heredity).

Fertilizers may influence the mineral composition of plants. The iodine content of a plant, for example, may vary with the iodine content of the soil, and the same may be true of other elements such as zinc, cobalt and selenium.

The fact that mineral content of soil can affect mineral content of its plants encourages the organic food industry to suggest that its recommended fertilizers are the best way to supply minerals. *"After all,"* they say, *"we return to nature what belongs to nature—animals which eat plants nourished by soil return the elements to the soil via their manure—nothing is lost."* This, however, is faulty reasoning. If a soil is deficient in a nutrient, use of manure from animals fed from that soil is the surest way to guarantee that the nutrient will remain missing. The best way to insure proper plant growth is to determine by analysis what the soil needs and to add the needed chemicals. Manure is unlikely to give a deficient soil exactly what it needs.

At the New York State hearing, Dr. Schwartz was asked whether Rodale Press publications generally take the position that organic foods are nutritionally superior to regular foods. He replied, *"I don't think that organic foods are any different from the foods that we ordinarily eat. The thing we are talking about is the method of producing these foods."*

Even if its leaders publicly deny making claims of nutritional superiority, however, there is no question that the industry as a whole suggests to its customers that its methods nourish plants better and therefore will nourish people better. To quote further from investigator White's testimony:

> Q. *Did you find a pattern of representation existed among the stores which you visited as to the virtues of organic food?*
>
> A. *Yes, sir, the general consensus was that they were . . . more nutritious and that they would be healthier in the long run if consumed by an individual.*
>
> Q. *Were any examples given to you of what would happen if you purchased organic food in regard to illness, was that stressed?*
>
> A. *Yes, there were a few establishments who told me that if you are a little heavy, and you eat organically grown food, you might lose some weight or might be free of diabetes.*

"Additions of Organic Matter"

The implication suggested here is that organic matter *alone* conditions soil best for plants. It has long been standard agricultural practice to plow crop residues and "green manuring crops" back into the soil. This makes the soil easier to work and can improve the seed-bed for the coming crop. This practice works well in combination with the use of fertilizers. Composts and animal manures may also help the physical characteristics of the soil. In fact, there are times when the so-called "mulching" process is needed and highly advantageous. Scientific farmers can easily determine and use whatever their soil needs. [Incidentally, plants can be grown "hydroponically," with no soil at all, with just chemical nutrients added to water. This is not yet practical for large-scale farming, but it highlights the lack of logic in the above "organic" myth.]

Low availability and high distribution costs make it clear that the world cannot rely upon animal-produced fertilizers to grow its food. It takes 20 pounds of manure to supply the same amount of nutrients as one pound of synthetic fertilizer. More often than not, the wastes from cows, horses and chickens accumulate at great distances from food-growing areas. It is expensive to collect and haul manures great distances and then spread them on the fields.

Manure has another disadvantage. It can contaminate plants with Salmonella germs which can cause serious diarrheal illness (dysentery). Manure can also spread intestinal parasites.

"Not Treated with Preservatives, Hormones, Antibiotics"

Here, the organic and health food promoters suggest that *all* "food additives" are "bad." But they do not tell you that without the use of additives, it would not be possible to feed large populations. They also omit mention that preservatives have been used for centuries to prevent foods from spoiling. The salting of meat and the pickling of cucumbers are familiar examples. Hormones are present naturally in *all* animals and plants. Antibiotics are not used to treat foods, but are valuable in controlling diseases of farm animals—some of which diseases are dangerous to humans. Some antibiotics which are fed to farm animals travel through their intestines without getting into their meat. Those that do get into the meat are destroyed by cooking.

131

Calcium propionate, which is used to prevent bread from getting moldy, offers another penetrating illustration of the health food industry's lack of logic about additives. Calcium propionate is normally produced as well as used in the human body. Leaving it out of bread will do the consumer no good whatsoever. It will, however, result in a lot of moldy bread being thrown in the garbage—at a time of food shortages and high prices. (And, as Dr. Herbert points out in Chapter 8, people who eat a Swiss cheese sandwich consume enough calcium propionate from the natural cheese to preserve two loaves of bread.)

These inconsistencies should make it clear that the health food industry's sweeping general attack on food additives does not make sense. The only proper way to evaluate food additives is to do so individually. Scientists do this, of course. FDA scientists, for example, set careful tolerance levels in foods and conduct frequent "market basket" studies wherein foods from 18 regions of the United States are purchased and analyzed.

"Etc."

The term "etc." is not defined. Presumably, this allows the definition to be expanded at will to keep pace with the imagination of "organic" producers. As Investigator White indicated at the Lefkowitz hearing, the "organic" label is not confined to fruits and vegetables:

> Q. *Did any specific food example stick in your mind, Mr. White?*
> A. *Yes, the eggs. I asked in several establishments why it is necessary to charge the inflated price for the eggs and I was told that these eggs were produced by organically grown chickens, that these chickens were free of hormones and they were allowed to roam free with the rooster and*

132

that's the reason why they had to charge the prices they are charging for the eggs.

Q. *Did you come upon a store that was selling fish?*

A. *Yes . . .*

Q. *Did the man selling fish tell you why it was organic?*

A. *Yes, he claimed that it was caught in the pollution-free, mineral-rich Atlantic Ocean.*

Q. *Did he have a sign to that effect, Mr. White?*

A. *Yes, he had a sign. I took a picture of that sign after interviewing that gentleman in the store.*

Taste

There are three factors which affect the taste of fruits and vegetables: (1) their genetic make-up; (2) how ripe they are when harvested; and (3) how fresh they are when eaten. "Organic" food advocates claim that their products taste better. They claim that since their produce comes from small farms, it is more likely to be sold locally in fresh condition. They also claim that supermarket produce is bred for shipping and keeping qualities rather than for flavor.

These claims were scientifically tested by research at the University of Florida. In this experiment, 20 men and women, ages 18 to 60, met several times a week for three months to compare 25 "health" foods with their supermarket cousins. Color, flavor, texture, odor and general acceptance were rated. None of the "health" foods was found to be superior on the basis of general acceptance. However, many of the regular foods were rated as better for color, flavor, texture and general acceptance. Regular foods that were scored higher than

133

health foods by the panel included dried apples, apple juice, applesauce, cashews, cereal, Swiss cheese, coconut, corn chips, ice cream, mayonnaise with tomato, peanut butter, sesame chips and tomato juice. The only health food qualities which were scored higher than those of regular foods were the odors of apple butter and pizza and the color of ketchup.

It is, of course, possible that some batches of "organically grown" foods will taste better than some conventionally grown foods. The point to keep in mind about this, however, is that superior taste will not be the result of organic methods, but of better heredity, better harvesting time or quicker marketing time.

Cost

Many studies have shown that foods labeled "organic" cost more than conventionally grown foods. In 1972, for example, the U.S. Department of Agriculture compared prices in the District of Columbia. Here is what they found:

Comparison of Regular and "Organic" Food Prices

| | SUPERMARKET | | HEALTH | NATURAL |
	"Regular" Department	"Organic" Department	Food Store	Food Store
Canned apple juice, qt.	.29	.65	.75	.51
Dried peaches, lb.	.73	1.32	1.68	1.55
Corn meal, lb.	.14	.30	.44	.21
Honey, lb.	.55	.79	1.05	.50
Cucumbers, lb.	.19	.79	.69	.57
Total of above 5 items	1.90	3.85	4.61	3.34
"Market basket" of 29 standard foods	11.00	20.30	21.90	17.80

The low prices of the regular supermarket foods are out of the Good Old Days. However, the most interesting thing about the table is the difference in price between regular and "organic" foods in the same super-

134

market. What do you think an on-the-ball store manager would do if he ran out of organic cucumbers and had plenty of the regular variety on hand (especially if he were aware that there is basically no difference between the two products anyway)?

The Appeal for "Consumer Protection"

Without a doubt, the typical 50–100% mark-up has led many enterprising merchants to label regular food as "organic." Calling this practice a "fraud," promoters of "real" organic food are asking our government to "protect" their customers from "fake" organic food. Ignoring the fact that "real" organic food is identical or inferior to regular food, they suggest that their customers should be able to get "what they *think* they are paying for"—that is, foods produced by "genuine" organic methods.

Rodale Press has designed a "certification" program whereby farmers who follow its suggested methods are given labels which indicate that their methods have met Rodale standards. Once the labels are given to the farmers, however, there is no practical way to supervise how the labels are used.

Organic certification proposals could be regarded as quite humorous except for the fact that some government officials have taken them seriously. Certification programs have actually been started in Oregon and New Hampshire. Not only that, but in Texas, the U.S. Office of Economic Opportunity is offering technical assistance so that "poor farmers can raise their incomes enough through organic farming to stay on the land."

Overview

Two hundred years ago, the average family in the Western world had to spend most of its time grubbing a meager living from the soil. The lack of fertilizer, the presence of pests that demolished crops, and the absence of knowledge about plant breeding all combined to keep most people hungry. Then chemists discovered that plants were actually nourished by inorganic chemicals. Phosphate, potash, nitrate and ammonia were needed. They could come either from the breakdown of manure by soil bacteria, or from rock phosphate, inorganic potash, nitrates and ammonia salts. The agricultural revolution was on. Farmers became able to feed more and more city folk.

A century ago, farmers were helpless against the fungus blight which turned their potatoes into a black slime. As a result, one million people starved to death during the Irish potato famine. Pesticides to control the blight were not yet available.

As agricultural knowledge increased by leaps and bounds, farming became increasingly scientific. Plant and animal breeding gave us fine new strains of grains, vegetables, fruits, poultry, pigs and cattle. More efficient fertilizers and a wide variety of pesticides were developed. Rare delicacies became commonplace.

The new chemical methods required careful regulation to see that farmers used them properly. Pure food laws were passed to make sure that only insignificant traces of unwanted pesticide residues were present in foods. These laws appear to be working well. There has not been one case of illness in America which can be attributed to a scientific agricultural procedure. In contrast, in countries where "organic" fertilizers (such as human waste) are used, food poisoning from disease organisms is quite common.

Against this 200 year background of fantastic scientific progress have emerged voices of quackery who cry that our food supply is neither safe nor nutritious. They either ignore or fail to understand scientific thought. They profit greatly by frightening the public into buying their ideas, their publications and their overpriced or unnecessary "health" products.

Many Americans, worried about pollution and flooded with misleading information in talk shows and publications, are responding to the quacks. Despite the fact that "organic food" cannot be defined, and despite the fact that foods labeled "organic" cannot be told apart from "regular" foods, people are willing to pay more for them. Americans now spend an estimated 500 million dollars a year for them.

But the ultimate irony is that the organic food industry, which itself preys on confusion and false hopes, is asking government to certify its fakery. With such legal approval, its customers would be purchasing "genuine" fakes.

The organic food lobby is clever and well-organized. Let us hope that government officials who are pressured by this lobby can see clearly who needs protection and from whom. Instead of protecting an industry which is itself a fake, our government should educate consumers. And since the "organic" label cannot be accurately defined, its commercial use should be outlawed.

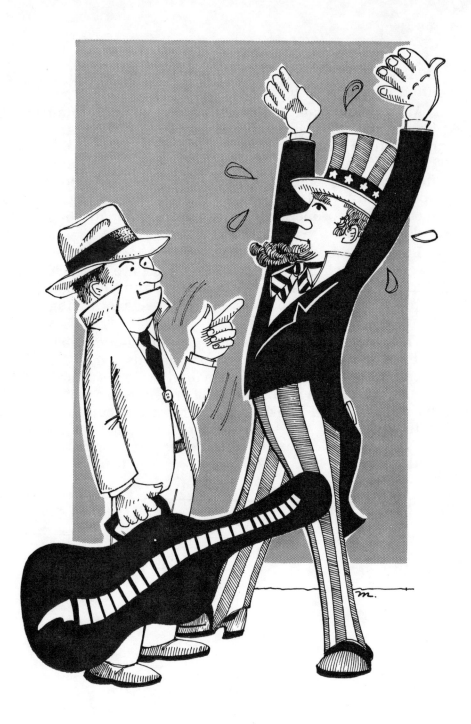

10

THE SPINE SALESMEN

". . . criteria which should be used by chiropractors when determining whether a patient is or is not a chiropractic case:
1. determine if the person has a spinal column
2. determine if the patient has a nervous system
3. determine if the patient is living."

— Douglas B. Gates, D.C.
Dean of Continuing Education
Sherman College of Chiropractic
Sherman Report, *1975*

BY

STEPHEN BARRETT, M.D.
Chairman, Board of Directors
Lehigh Valley Committee Against Health Fraud, Inc.

Harriet Cressman is a lovely lady who lives with her husband on their farm in Pleasant Valley, Pennsylvania. Early in 1963, she developed a backache. Thinking that chiropractors were "bone specialists," she went to one. He did not disappoint her. After examining her and taking an x-ray, he said that her spine was "tilted" but could be corrected by spinal "adjustments." The adjustments took place three times a week for several months. As her back symptoms improved, her treatment was reduced to twice a week, then once a week and then once a month. At this point, although Harriet felt completely well, the chiropractor suggested that she continue adjustments regularly for "preventive maintenance." She did so faithfully for ten years and had no further trouble with her back—as far as she knew. In November 1973, however, the chiropractor took another x-ray and gave her bad news: the x-ray showed "18 compressed discs and progressive osteoarthritis of the spine which was spreading rapidly." It would make her a helpless cripple if she did not have immediate treatment. He reassured her, however, that his new machinery could correct her disc problem and stop the spread of her arthritis.

Staggered by the news, Harriet went home to discuss the matter with her husband. But the chiropractor's receptionist had already telephoned Mr. Cressman to ask him to bring Harriet back immediately to the office. Because of the serious nature of the case, the chiropractor wished to begin "intensive treatment" that same day. The treatment would be in day-long sessions, alternating complete bed rest with "Diapulse" and "Anatomotor" therapy, spinal adjustments and acupuncture. Its cost would be $11,000, but with payment in advance, the doctor would accept an even $10,000.

Because of her long association with the chiropractor,

and because she was in no mood to trifle about her health, she unhesitatingly went about raising the money. Supplementing her life savings with a bank loan, she paid in advance.

For the next few months, as far as she could tell, Harriet's treatment proceeded smoothly. Every week another full spine x-ray was taken. Each time the chiropractor pointed out on the x-ray how she improved. He also discussed other patients with her and asked her to help talk them into treatment with him. Advising Harriet that her condition might be hereditary, he suggested that other members of her family have spinal x-rays.

Harriet's son Donald did have an x-ray and was told by the chiropractor that he had a "pin dot of arthritis which, if untreated, would spread like wildfire and leave him crippled within a short time." Donald's cost? With the usual ten percent discount for advance payment—a mere $1,500!

In May, 1974, the chiropractor suddenly informed the Cressmans that he was moving to California. "What about us?" they asked. "Don't worry," he answered, but their worry increased and turned to suspicion when his answers became contradictory. Pressed by Harriet for the name of another chiropractor who could continue her treatment, the chiropractor named one. "Don't bother to call him before I leave," he said, "because he has already gone over your records and x-rays with me." Harriet did contact her chiropractor-to-be, however, and was told that her name had been "mentioned" but that no record or x-ray review had taken place.

Shocked by the turn of events, the Cressmans consulted medical and legal authorities who suggested that they file criminal charges for "theft by deception." They did. Investigation by the Northampton County

141

District Attorney's office uncovered other patients of the chiropractor who had similar experiences. A medical radiologist x-rayed the spines of Harriet and Donald and offered to testify at trial that neither had any condition which could possibly be helped by chiropractic treatment. When news of the arrest became public, a third patient filed a criminal complaint. The chiropractor, he claimed, had cheated him out of $2,075 by promising to cure his arm and leg which had been paralyzed by a "stroke."

Now it was the chiropractor's turn to be stunned by the turn of events. He disappeared from public view and communicated through his attorney. He was innocent, he claimed, but was anxious to leave Pennsylvania as soon as possible. [He could not do so until the criminal cases were settled.] If the three complainants would drop their charges, he would return their money. Under supervision of the Northampton County Court, the $13,575 was returned and the charges were dropped.

Do you wonder whether Harriet Cressman had to be very gullible in order to part with $10,000 for such questionable treatment? Please let me assure you that she is a very intelligent person who is not at all gullible. *Until the chiropractor announced that he was leaving, she simply had no reason to be suspicious.* Though generally well-informed, she had never encountered criticism of chiropractic in any newspaper, magazine, book or radio or television program. Like all chiropractors, hers was licensed by the State *as a doctor.* He seemed warm, friendly and genuinely interested in Harriet. And he did what she would expect a doctor to do. He examined her, took an x-ray, made a "diagnosis" and prescribed a "treatment" plan. She was happy to feel better and, like most people, gave no thought to whether the "treatment" had cured her or whether she would have recovered just as quickly with no treatment at all. Nor did she give any thought to the nature of chiropractic itself, how it began, how its practitioners are trained or what they usually do. She certainly did not suspect that chiropractic is based on the mistaken beliefs of a grocer and his son.

The Development of Chiropractic

Chiropractic claims it began in 1895 when Daniel David Palmer restored the hearing of a deaf janitor by "adjusting" a bump on his spine. Palmer thought he had helped the man by releasing pressure on the nerve to his ear. A grocer and "magnetic healer" by profession, he did not know that the nerve from the brain to the ear does not travel inside the spinal column. But no matter—he soon became certain that he had discovered *the* cause of disease.

At first he kept the "discovery" secret, but by the end of 1895 he set up the Palmer College of Chiropractic to teach it. One of his early pupils was his own son, Bartlett Joshua, better known as "B. J." The boy began to help his father run the school soon after it opened. Gradually, however, B. J. took over. In 1906, Daniel David was charged with practicing medicine without a license and went to jail. When he was released, B. J. bought out his interest in the school. Business boomed, and many Palmer graduates opened schools of their own. Cash was the basic entrance requirement for most of them and some even trained their students by mail.

As competition among chiropractors grew, and as many were jailed for practicing medicine without a license, they began to pressure state legislators to license them. Responding to this pressure, perhaps with the hope that licensing would lead to higher standards of education and practice, states began to pass licensing laws. Chiropractors would be allowed no drugs or surgery. Most states limited chiropractic treatment to "spinal adjustment." *But for what?* If all disease was caused by spines which need adjustment, couldn't chiropractors treat everything?

They could. And they did. Over the years, many cases have come to light where chiropractors treated patients for cancer and other serious diseases which should have had medical attention.

The Scope of "Modern" Chiropractic

Does this mean that no matter what is wrong with you, if you go to a chiropractor today, he will diagnose your problem as a "pinched nerve" and want to treat you with spinal adjustments? According to chiropractic officials, the modern chiropractor most often treats musculoskeletal problems such as backaches and stiff necks. In 1974, Stephen Owens, D.C., Past-President of the American Chiropractic Association, was asked by *Medical Economics* magazine what chiropractors do. Said Owens: "A chiropractor would be silly to take on a disease that's not susceptible to his kind of treatment. He'd just be inviting failure."

Owens' statement was similar to what chiropractors told Congress as they lobbied for Medicare inclusion. In 1970, for example, William Day, D.C., President of the International Chiropractors Association, was questioned by U.S. Senate Finance Committee Chairman Russell Long:

> Long: The medical profession says that your profession claims to treat all sorts of things for which it can do no good whatever.
>
> Day: Let me state categorically that the chiropractor does not claim to be able to cure all conditions . . .

Long: How about migraine?
Day: No.
Long: You don't treat ulcers?
Day: No, sir.
Long: What about hepatitis?
Day: Hepatitis is an infectious disease. We would refer it to a physician.

Such answers from top chiropractic officials sound quite reasonable and easy to believe. After all, who nowadays could accept Palmer's original belief that all disease had just one cause or that one method of treatment can cure everything? But many studies suggest that official chiropractic is not willing to admit what chiropractors are actually doing.

In 1963 the American Chiropractic Association asked its members what conditions they treated. Of those responding, 85% said that they treated musculoskeletal conditions most frequently. However, the following percentages reported treating other conditions:

Asthma	89%	Pneumonia	32%
Gallbladder	82%	Acute heart	
Ulcers	76%	conditions	31%
Chronic heart condition	70%	Appendicitis	30%
Tonsillitis	67%	Pernicious anemia	24%
Impaired hearing	59%	Cerebral hemorrhage	18%
Goiter	48%	Fractures	9%
Diabetes mellitus	46%	Leukemia	8%
Rheumatic fever	37%	Cancer	7%
Hepatitis	32%	Diphtheria	4%

In 1971, skeptical about Dr. Day's testimony, the Lehigh Valley Committee Against Health Fraud sent the following inquiry to 130 members of his organization selected at random from its Directory:

"I have been suffering from ulcers and sometimes migraine headaches for many years. I

145

am going to this chiropractor near my home now and he is helping me. But I am not finished treatments and my husband has a job near you. Do you treat these conditions? Do you think I can finish my treatments with you?"

Of the 110 who replied, 75% offered treatment and the rest offered welcome without directly answering the questions about treatment. Not one said no. A similar letter asked 92 other chiropractors whether they treated hepatitis. Only one of 72 who replied answered negatively—that he might not be able to take the case because his state law required reporting of communicable disease. However, another chiropractor from the same state said that "chiropractic offers the safest and best care for hepatitis, as well as many other conditions."

In 1973 Dr. Murray Katz, a Canadian pediatrician, surveyed chiropractic offices in Ottawa, Canada. Seven out of nine displayed pamphlets which exaggerated what chiropractors can do. When a chiropractic official responded that use of such pamphlets would cause automatic 30-day license suspension, Katz noted that no chiropractor had ever been suspended for their use.

Additional evidence that chiropractors do not know their limitations comes from advertising. The Lehigh Valley Committee Against Health Fraud has collected hundreds of chiropractic ads which contain false claims. Among them:

"There are very few diseases . . . which are not treatable by chiropractic methods."

"Diabetes . . . the chief cause lies in displaced spinal vertebrae . . ."

"Question: If a surgeon cuts out a tumor of the stomach, does he not remove the cause?
Answer: No, he may have removed the cause

146

of the distress in the stomach, but he has not removed the cause of the tumor and it will probably grow again. A chiropractor adjusts the cause of the tumor."

"If every person were under regular chiropractic care, the incidence of cancer would be reduced by 50% in ten years."

"There is hardly an illness that does not respond to chiropractic care."

During the past six years, I have collected chiropractic journals and textbooks, listened to chiropractic lectures, spoken and corresponded with hundreds of chiropractors and interviewed many of their patients. My effort to define the scope of chiropractic has led me to three conclusions:

1) Many chiropractors do not know their limitations.

2) What chiropractors say about what they do depends greatly upon who they think is listening.

3) *Chiropractors themselves are confused and cannot agree about either what they are actually doing or what they should be doing.*

There are undoubtedly some chiropractors who make a sincere effort to quickly refer people who need medical attention to an appropriate physician. Doing this well, however, requires a good medical education.

Which brings us to the question of what chiropractors learn in school.

Chiropractic Education

If D. D. Palmer could look at current chiropractic schools, he would be surprised. In his day, chiropractic training lasted two weeks to one year and covered just spinal analysis and treatment. Today, chiropractic school takes four years and includes many subjects which Palmer would think were not related to his

147

"great discovery." Among these are "basic sciences" such as anatomy, biochemistry, bacteriology and pathology, and clinical subjects such as psychiatry, study of x-ray, obstetrics (delivery of babies) and pediatrics. Standard medical textbooks are used in many of these courses.

There are several reasons for these changes. As licensing laws became stricter, many states required testing in basic sciences. Chiropractic schools which could not prepare their students for these exams could not remain in business, and an estimated 600 of them have closed. Thirteen schools exist today.

Because Palmer's basic theory is false, chiropractic has been under continual attack from the scientific community. Since few people nowadays could believe that all diseases have just one cause or cure, many chiropractors have modified their philosophies. "Modern" chiropractic, its leaders claim, recognizes the value of modern medicine and refers patients who need medical care to proper physicians. "Modern" chiropractors, their leaders claim, recognize that factors such as germs and hormones play a role in disease. "We would like to work together," they say. "While the medical doctor gives antibiotics to kill germs or insulin to control diabetes, we will eliminate pinched nerves so the body can heal itself."

Unfortunately, despite the "new" look of chiropractic education, close observation suggests that much of it is a hoax. In 1960, for example, the Stanford (Calif.) Research Institute published a study which included inspection of two chiropractic schools. They noted that although certain scientific subjects were part of the school programs, the school libraries and laboratories did not appear to be in actual use.

In 1963, the AMA Department of Investigation sent applications from nonexistent persons who did not appear to meet admission requirements listed in chiropractic school catalogues. Only two out of seven were rejected.

In 1966, the AMA published a study of the educational backgrounds of teachers at chiropractic schools. Fewer than half had graduated from college and many who taught basic sciences did not even have degrees in the subjects they taught. When I examined current catalogues four years later, I found that little had changed. Since that time, some chiropractic schools have affiliated with nearby colleges so that students can get training in basic sciences from properly trained instructors. Other chiropractic schools have added teachers who have degrees in these subjects. But neither of these changes will greatly increase the quality of chiropractic training. Basic science courses merely prepare students for the *study* of disease. They do not prepare them to make diagnoses or prescribe treatment.

In 1968, a large-scale study by the U.S. Department of Health, Education and Welfare concluded that "chiropractic education does not prepare its practitioners to make adequate diagnoses or to provide appropriate treatment." The HEW Report quotes many chiropractic statements which helped to bring about this conclusion. Among them:

> "For the chiropractor, diagnosis does not constitute, as it does for the medical doctor, a specific guide for treatment . . ."
>
> *Opportunities in A Chiropractic Career,* 1967
> Prepared by American Chiropractic Association
> and International Chiropractors Association

> ". . . chiropractic adjusting is efficacious in handling both the acute and chronic cases of coronary occlusion . . ."

149

Neurodynamics of Vertebral Subluxation, 1962 by A. E. Homewood, D.C. (the most widely used chiropractic textbook).

"Q. Do you think that if an acute appendicitis was identified early enough in the disease process, chiropractic can cure it?

A. Yes I do. I say this strictly from experience. I don't say it only from my experience but from the experience of all who practice."

1968 testimony of H. R. Frogley, D.C.
Dean of Academic Affairs, Palmer College of Chiropractic.

Chiropractic attacked the HEW Report as "biased," and implied that HEW failed to look at "modern" chiropractic. Considering that the Report was based primarily upon information submitted by leading chiropractic organizations, these charges seem odd. Actually, they are true to form. *Whenever chiropractic is attacked by an outsider, it claims its attacker is "biased." Whenever it is embarrassed by quotes from within its own profession, it claims they are not representative.*

How Dangerous Is Chiropractic?

It should be obvious that to help you, doctors must first be able to figure out what is wrong with you. Yet chiropractors who believe that spinal problems cause all diseases may not even *try* to make medical diagnoses. According to Reginald Gold, D.C., "If you were to come to my office, I wouldn't want to know what is wrong with you. I wouldn't want to know what your symptoms are. I would want to do one thing . . . examine your spine." Gold said this at a public meeting in 1971 after a colleague introduced him as "one of the country's leading authorities on chiropractic" and a lecturer on the faculty of three chiropractic schools. Currently, he is Vice-President of Development of the Sherman College of Chiropractic.

Although many chiropractors share Gold's philosophy, the majority probably do try to determine whether their patients need medical treatment. Most patients protect themselves from misdiagnosis by consulting medical doctors before they go to chiropractors. Those who start with chiropractors, of course, take a greater risk. Not only are chiropractors poorly trained to make diagnoses, but they are prohibited by law from doing some tests which may be crucial to medical investigation.

Although spinal manipulation has a small place in the treatment of back disorders, in the hands of chiropractors it can be dangerous. I know of one man who was paralyzed from the waist down after a spinal manipulation. Unknown to his chiropractor, spinal cancer had weakened the patient's spinal bones so that the treatment had crushed his spinal cord. In another case I investigated, a patient who took anticoagulants (blood thinners) had serious bleeding into his back muscles after a manipulation. Surgery was required to remove the collected blood.

From time to time, broken bones, paralyses and strokes have been noted in court cases and medical journals. So have deaths from cancer and infectious diseases where chiropractors did not know enough to make medical referral in time for proper medical treatment. Although such serious cases are relatively rare, they are inexcusable. Lesser complications such as sprains are more common, but statistics are hard to collect. Some patients are too embarrassed to publicize them. Some do not realize that their extra discomfort is the result of inappropriate treatment. And others are sufficiently fond of their chiropractor that they cannot believe he has mistreated them.

151

X-ray by chiropractors are a leading source of unnecessary radiation. A full-spine x-ray exposes sexual
organs to from 10 to 1,000 times as much radiation as a
routine chest x-ray. This is dangerous because it can
lead to increased numbers of birth defects in future
generations. Most chiropractors use x-rays. A 1971 survey of the *Journal of Clinical Chiropractic* suggests
that more than ten million x-rays were taken each year
by U.S. and Canadian chiropractors. Of these, two million were the 14 × 36 inch full-spine type. Chiropractic
inclusion under Medicare, which began in July 1973,
will probably increase these numbers greatly.

Chiropractors claim that x-rays help them locate the
"subluxations" which D. D. Palmer imagined were the
cause of "pinched nerves" and "nerve interference."
But they do not agree among themselves about what
subluxations are. Some chiropractors believe that subluxations are displaced bones which can be seen on
x-rays and can be put back in place by spinal adjustments. Other chiropractors define subluxations
vaguely and insist that they do not show on x-rays. But
what chiropractors say about x-rays also depends upon
who asks.

When the National Association of Letter Carriers
Health Plan included chiropractic, it received claims
for treatment of cancer, heart disease, mumps, mental
retardation and many other questionable conditions. In
1964, chiropractors were asked to justify such claims
by sending x-ray evidence of spinal problems. They
submitted hundreds, all of which were supposed to
show subluxations. When chiropractic officials were
asked to review them, however, they were unable to
point out a single subluxation.

Some chiropractic textbooks show "before and after"
x-rays which are supposed to demonstrate subluxations. In 1971, to get a closer look at such x-rays, our

Committee challenged the Lehigh Valley Chiropractic Society to demonstrate ten sets. They refused, suggesting instead that we ask the Palmer School to show us some from its "teaching files." When we did, however, Ronald Frogley, D.C., replied, "Chiropractors do not make the claim to be able to read a specific subluxation from an x-ray film."

Frogley might have answered more cautiously had he anticipated the wording by which Congress included chiropractic under Medicare. Payment would be made for treatment of "subluxations *demonstrated by x-rays to exist.*" To help chiropractors get paid, the American Chiropractic Association has issued a *Basic Chiropractic Procedural Manual* which defines subluxations as anything which can interfere with spinal function and says, "Since we are obligated to find subluxations before receiving payment, it behooves us to make an objective study of what films show in the way of subluxations . . ." Referring to the Letter Carriers experience as "an unfortunate debacle which almost destroyed chiropractic credibility in Washington," it cautions, in italics, *"The subluxations must be perfectly obvious and indisputable."*

If a chiropractor limited his practice to muscular conditions such as simple backaches, if he saw patients only on referral from medical doctors after medical diagnosis has been made, if he were not overly vigorous in his manipulations, if he consulted and referred to medical doctors when he couldn't handle a problem, and if he avoided the use of x-rays, his patients might be relatively safe. But he might not be able to earn a living.

The Selling of the Spine

A chiropractor's income depends not only on what he treats but on how well he can sell himself. The American Chiropractic Association estimates that the "average" chiropractor earns about $31,000 per year, but the meaning of this figure is not clear. Many chiropractic graduates do not remain in practice and others are forced to practice part-time. Top chiropractic salesmen can earn a fortune.

Intensive selling of the spine begins in chiropractic school as instructors convey the scope and philosophy of chiropractic to their students. Chiropractic graduates can get help from many practice-building consultants, the most expensive of which is Clinic Masters. In 1973, Clinic Masters estimated that 15,000 chiropractors practiced actively in the United States and Canada and said it represented more than 1,800 of them. Its fee is $10,000—$100 on entrance and the rest payable as income rises. In 1973 its directors said, "many of our clients have moved right on up through the $50,000, $100,000, $150,000 income levels to $300,000 and above" and that "before long practice incomes of $500,000 will not be rare."

Clinic Masters promotes the idea that higher income means greater service to patients. Such service includes charging for each adjustment or other unit of treatment instead of a flat office fee, an overall "case" fee instead of charging per visit, and "intensive care," which adds room or ward fees to the bill. In 1974, 132 of its clients reported charging an average of $129.43 per day for intensive care.

Clinic Masters apparently wants the details of its advice to remain a private matter. Its clients sign a secrecy agreement and new applicants are checked against directory lists to make sure that they really are chiropractors. It also offers a $10,000 reward to anyone who is first to report "disparaging statements about Clinic Masters or its clients" which lead to a successful lawsuit.

The largest practice-building firm appears to be the

154

Parker Chiropractic Research Foundation of Fort Worth, Texas. Its founder, James W. Parker, D.C., claims that "more than 13,000 chiropractors, wives and assistants" have attended his four-day courses. Unlike Clinic Masters, Parker has not been cautious about revealing his techniques to outsiders. In 1968, an investigative reporter named Ralph Lee Smith gained admission to Parker's course by pretending to be a chiropractor and paying its $250 fee. Emerging with a diploma that he had "completed the prescribed course of study at the Parker Chiropractic Research Seminar," Smith published what he observed.

Parker's course is built around a 335-page *Textbook of Office Procedure and Practice Building for the Chiropractic Profession*. Parker appears to believe that the scope of chiropractic is unlimited. The *Textbook* suggests that patients be offered a "free consultation" but led into an "examination" which costs them money. It suggests that "One adjustment for each year of age is a rough thumbnail guide of what people will willingly accept and pay for," but "If in doubt about the payment or the return of the patient, take only the smaller x-rays on the first visit but ostensibly x-ray fully."

Share International, Parker's sales organization, sells a wide variety of practice-building aids. One is a chart which pictures a spine and claims that more than 100 diseases are related to nerve pressure at its various parts. Included are: hernias, appendicitis, crossed eyes, diabetes, anemia, gallbladder conditions, hardening of the arteries and thyroid conditions.

For about $20, chiropractors can get copies of 107 advertisements to "guide" preparation of their own ads. Most of the ads are case histories, and the instructions which accompany them suggest: "Re-type each ad on your own stationery for presentation to the editor. This would indicate that they are your own creations, and

that the cases mentioned . . . are from your own files."
For about $45, graduates of Parker's basic course can
purchase a set of ten cassette tapes which give additional advice. In *Sentences that Sell,* Parker describes
how chiropractors associated with him test ideas scientifically and report back to him how they work. In *Ways
to Stimulate Referrals,* he tells how to steer conversations to sick people. "In a casual, natural way," patients should be asked about the health of their
families, friends and neighbors. Should any be ailing,
patients should be urged to be "Good Samaritans" by
telling them about "all the wonderful things" that
chiropractic might do for them.

Despite his questionable methods, Parker appears to
be a highly respected and integral part of the chiropractic world. He is a welcome lecturer at chiropractic
schools. In fact, in 1970, when one of my Committee
members merely requested a catalogue from the Texas
Chiropractic College, he received a letter from Parker
telling how chiropractors often reach incomes of $50–
$100,000 per year.

Sid Williams, D.C., of Atlanta, Georgia, is another
leading promoter. His many enterprises include a
chiropractic supply house, several publications,
practice-building courses, and the recently opened Life
Chiropractic College. According to a College booklet,
"thousands" of chiropractors follow his philosophy.
Known as Life Fellows, they appear to believe that virtually all conditions should be treated by chiropractic
methods. His practice-building techniques appear to
stress mass-production. Ads for his seminars boast that
their top instructors see 600 to 1,000 patients per week.
And at a 1973 hearing for deceptive advertising, one
Life Fellow testified that he "adjusted" 593 patients in
a single day!

Many chiropractors recommend regular "preventive

maintenance" to increase resistance and prolong life. Reginald Gold, for example, hopes that "every man, woman and child will see his chiropractor once a week for life" so that they can live "120 to 150 years." Other chiropractors have told me that all people, sick or well, should have regular chiropractic care. Wondering what approach chiropractors would take toward healthy people, our Committee once sent a perfectly well four-year old girl to five chiropractors for a "check-up." The first said the child's shoulder blades were "out of place" and found "pinched nerves to her stomach and gallbladder." The second said the child's pelvis was "twisted." The third said one hip was "elevated" and that spinal misalignments could cause "headaches, nervousness, equilibrium or digestive problems" in the future. The fourth predicted "bad periods and rough childbirth" if her "shorter left leg" were not treated. The fifth not only found hip and neck problems, but also "adjusted" them without bothering to ask permission. Unfortunately, the adjustments were so painful that we decided to end our experiment.

Chiropractic has been described as the "greatest tribute to applied public relations that the world has ever known." Despite its shortcomings, millions of people have tried it. Chiropractic's ultimate goal is inclusion in national health insurance. And unless concerned citizens can find ways to organize and protest, your tax dollars will wind up paying for D. D. Palmer's dreams.

Overview

In 1895, modern medicine was in its infancy. Many of its theories were just as ridiculous as that of Palmer. Since that time, medicine has become a science. Chiropractic, however, has not. The only science chiropractic has developed is that of salesmanship.

157

Chiropractors, of course, will deny this. They will say that since I am "biased," this chapter is deliberately slanted to make them look bad. But what I have reported comes mainly from its schools, its organizations, its recognized leaders and its official publications. My data truly represent chiropractic as it is today.

This book will tell you about many practitioners who have gained large and faithful followings even though their theories make no sense at all. Such practitioners rely upon salesmanship and the fact that most people get better without treatment.

Chiropractors win many friends with their warm manner, their seductive techniques, and their physical therapy and massage. But *going to a chiropractor is a distinct gamble*.

Recommended Reading

At Your Own Risk: The Case Against Chiropractic, by Ralph Lee Smith

Bonesetting, Chiropractic and Cultism, by Samuel Homola

11

THE POISONMONGERS

*More than 10,000 scientific studies attest to fluoridation's safety and effectiveness in preventing tooth decay . . .
Don't let the poisonmongers scare you.*

BY

MARY BERNHARDT
Secretary, Council on Dental Health
American Dental Association
and
BOB SPRAGUE

On May 27, 1975, 213,573 people in Los Angeles exercised their democratic privilege—*and voted against healthier teeth!* Since 1973, more than 270 Nebraska communities have done the same. In cities from coast to coast, citizens have voted to deprive themselves, their children, and their neighbors' children of the proven health benefits of fluoridation.

Of course, none of these negative voters meant to inflict cavities upon anyone. They were confused—influenced by alarmists who claim that adding fluoride to a city's water supply will "poison" people.

These alarmists are the "poisonmongers." Antagonistic to scientific research, they are commonly known as "antis" (short for "antifluoridationists"). Leaders of the 30-year struggle for fluoridation are frustrated by their tactics. Newspaper editors are commonly taken in by their publicity stunts. And legislators are often overwhelmed by their various and sometimes shrill arguments.

G. Herbert Seberg, D.D.S., knows the antis well. Past-President of the Nebraska Dental Association, he has been fighting to fluoridate Nebraska since 1950. In 1973, Dr. Seberg received two awards for his work in gaining passage of a bill which would order statewide fluoridation by January 1, 1975.

Promoting the bill, the Nebraska Dental Association led a five-month campaign which had the editorial support of most of the state's newspapers. Opposing the bill was the Nebraska Pure Air and Water Committee. Though loosely organized, its members distributed scare pamphlets, wrote letters to newspaper editors and paid for misleading advertisements.

Though the fluoridation bill passed, Dr. Seberg and his allies could not stem the dogged opposition of a few senators who attached an "escape clause" to it. Fifteen percent of a town's voters could petition for a referendum which would decide the fate of fluoridation in their community. By 1975, although 69 percent of Nebraska's one and one-half million people were drinking fluoridated water, more than 300 of its communities put the issue to a vote. Most of these were small, conservative prairie towns. Fewer than ten percent of these communities voted to fluoridate.

Los Angeles was the largest city ever to vote on this issue. Because of this, its referendum defeat was a great disappointment to fluoridation proponents. In September 1974, the Los Angeles City Council had voted 10–5 to fluoridate. But a few weeks later, pressure from frightened constituents persuaded the Council to allow the public to vote. After the referendum was defeated, 213,573 to 166,549, councilmen voted unanimously to rescind the fluoridation ordinance. Labeling the referendum defeat "a victory of strident scare tactics over medical evidence," a *Los Angeles Times* editorial criticized City Council for "retreating from its best judgment."

To date, more than 2,000 American communities have decided the matter of fluoridation at the voting booth. In thousands of other communities, the decision to fluoridate was made by city councils. In recent years, most voters have been rejecting fluoridation. Though this trend is discouraging, public health leaders are not surprised by it. As far back as 1951, Dr. Frank A. Bull, Director of Dental Education for the Wisconsin State Board of Health, summed up the problem quite well. Speaking at the Fourth Annual Conference of State Dental Directors, Dr. Bull said:

"I don't believe that you can win approval of any public health program where there is organized opposition. I mean clever, well thought-up opposition. I think it is possible to beat almost anything."

In the years since this statement was made, antifluoridationists have developed clever political tactics which can play on the fears of ordinary citizens. Increasingly, these tactics have been employed to bring about referenda—to defeat fluoridation. The sad fact is that people can easily be frightened by things which they do not understand and can easily be confused by contradictory arguments.

Fluoridation's Credentials

There should be no mystery about what fluoridation is. Fluoride is a mineral which occurs naturally in most water supplies. Fluoridation is the adjustment of the natural fluoride concentration to about one part of fluoride to one million parts of water. More than 10,000 scientific studies attest to fluoridation's safety and effectiveness in preventing tooth decay.

The history of fluoridation in the U.S. underlines its unique standing as a public health measure copied from a natural phenomenon. In the early 1900's, Dr. Frederick S. McKay began an almost 30-year search for the cause of the staining of teeth which was prevalent in Colorado where he practiced dentistry. Traveling to trace this condition, he found it common in other states, including Texas where it was known as "Texas teeth." In 1928, he announced that these teeth, although stained, showed "a singular absence of decay." He concluded that both the staining and the decay resistance were caused by something in the water. In 1931, the "something" was identified as fluoride.

The Public Health Service then took over to determine precisely what amount of fluoride in the water would prevent decay without causing staining. Years of "shoeleather epidemiology" by Dr. H. Trendley Dean traced the dental status of 7,000 children drinking naturally fluoridated water in 21 cities in four states. In

1943, he reported that the ideal amount of fluoride was one part per million parts of water. This concentration was demonstrated to result in healthy, attractive teeth which had one-third as many cavities as might otherwise be expected—and no staining. Dean, later known as the "father of fluoridation," thus paved the way for the control and public use of this natural phenomenon.

The next step was to determine whether water engineering could copy nature's amazing dental health benefit. At several test sites, the fluoride concentration of the public water supply was adjusted to one part per million.

One such test was conducted in the neighboring cities of Newburgh and Kingston, New York. First, the children in both cities were examined by dentists and physicians. Then fluoride was added to Newburgh's water supply. After ten years, the children of Newburgh had 58% fewer decayed teeth than those of unfluoridated Kingston. The greatest benefits were obtained by children who had drunk the fluoridated water since birth. Other studies showed that teeth made stronger by fluoride during childhood will remain permanently resistant to decay.

As the evidence for fluoridation piled up, thousands of communities acted to obtain its benefits. By 1975, more than 100 million Americans were drinking fluoridated water. But 100 million other Americans were receiving public water supplies which were not fluoridated—thanks largely to the efforts of poisonmongers.

Opposition to Fluoridation

Since it began, fluoridation has encountered opposition from scattered groups and individuals. Many of them have been associated with the health food industry—which aligns fluoridation with its general propaganda that our food supply is being "poisoned"

(see Chapter 8). Chiropractors have opposed fluoridation as an interference with "free choice of health
care." Christian Scientists have regarded it as "forced
medication" and the John Birch Society has seen it as a
"Communist plot."

By the early 1950's, individuals and local groups
began exchanging ideas and experiences with each
other. A few physicians and dentists became very vigorous in opposing fluoridation and began traveling
around the U.S. to appear at court hearings and public
meetings. One of them, George Waldbott, M.D., started
the *National Fluoridation News,* a four-page newspaper now edited by Mrs. Ethel Fabian of Gravette,
Arkansas.

Several national groups have been formed for the sole
purpose of fighting fluoridation, but it appears that
none of these has achieved sufficient funding to have
much impact outside of the communities of their leaders. However, several well-funded national multi-issue
organizations have managed to disseminate large
amounts of scare propaganda throughout the country.
Among them are Rodale Press (see Chapter 12), the
John Birch Society and the National Health Federation
(see Chapter 13).

The early efforts of the antifluoridationists were assisted by the caution and conservatism of many physicians, dentists and other scientists who felt that not
enough research had been done for them to take a positive stand. As time went on and data piled up, however,
the overwhelming majority of health scientists concluded that fluoridation is safe and effective.

But while scientists were refining and publishing
their experiments, the antis were refining and publishing their battle plans. In the mid-1960's, the National
Health Federation published *An Action Guide . . . On
How to Fight Fluoridation in Your Area.* Available for

25¢, this four-page leaflet details the strategy which can be used in any community where fluoridation is being considered.

"Neutralizing" Politicians

Once fluoridation proponents are known to be active, the leaflet says, antis should immediately send a letter to each member of governing bodies. The letter should emphasize "the most recent evidence" that fluoridation is "harmful." Most important, it should urge the officials to "remain absolutely neutral" by putting the matter to public vote. "When this is done," the leaflet states, "whatever political figures may be concerned are relieved of any and all responsibility in the matter."

This opening blast is designed to neutralize politicians. It aims to arouse doubt about the safety of fluoridation. It also offers an easy excuse for delaying favorable action—while the antis begin their hatchet job on public opinion.

How Poisonmongers Work

The antis' basic technique is *the big lie*. Made infamous by Hitler, it is simple to use, yet surprisingly effective. It consists of claiming that fluoridation causes cancer, heart disease, kidney disease and other serious ailments which people fear. The fact that there is no supporting evidence for such claims does not matter. The trick is to keep repeating them—because if something is said often enough, people tend to think there must be some truth to it.

A variation of the big lie is the *laundry list*. List enough "evils," and even if proponents can reply to some of them, they will never be able to cover the entire list. This technique is most effective in debates or letters to the editor.

165

A key factor in any anti campaign is the use of printed matter. Because of this, antis are very anxious to have their views printed in any publications. Scientific journals will rarely print them, but most local newspapers are sympathetic toward the expression of minority viewpoints regardless of whether they are supported by facts. A few editors even welcome the controversy the antis generate—on the theory that it will increase readership.

The aim of anti "documents" is to create the illusion of scientific controversy. Often they quote statements which are *out of date* or *out of context*. Quotes from obscure or hard-to-locate journals are particularly effective. Another favored tactic is to *misquote* a pro-fluoridation scientist, knowing that even if the scientist himself protests, his reply will not reach all of the people who saw the original misquote.

Half-truths are commonly used. For example, saying that fluoride is a rat poison ignores the fact that poison is a matter of dose. Large amounts of many substances—even pure water—can poison people. But the trace amount of fluoride contained in fluoridated water will not harm anyone.

"Experts" are commonly quoted. It is possible to find someone with scientific credentials who is against just about anything. Most "experts" who speak out against fluoridation, however, are not experts on the subject. There are, of course, a few dentists and physicians who oppose fluoridation. However, many of them oppose it on the basis of government action rather than on safety. Curiously, when anti experts change their minds in favor of fluoridation, they sometimes find that the antis keep on quoting their earlier positions.

Innuendo is a technique that has broad appeal because it can be used in a seemingly unemotional pitch. Some antis admit that fluoridation has been found safe

166

"so far," but claim that its long-range effects have "not yet" been fully explored. *The waiting game* is a related gambit in which antis suggest that waiting a bit longer will help to resolve "doubt" about fluoridation's safety. No doubt, some antis will continue to use this argument for a few hundred more years.

The *bogus reward* is a fascinating technique. Some antis offer large rewards to anyone who will prove that fluoridation is safe. If the wording is not extremely careful, however, the pros can actually collect. In 1965, a California chiropractor offered $1,000 to anyone who could produce an expert from California "who has done any conclusive research proving the safety" or who could produce documentary evidence that fluoridation is safe. A local dental group assembled a barrage of experts and more than 100 research reports testifying to fluoridation's safety and effectiveness. When the chiropractor refused to pay, the dental group filed suit and later settled out of court for $500.

A $100,000 reward offer has survived for a long time—but a close look will show why. In order to collect, pros must post a bond "to cover any costs which the offerers of the reward might incur if the proof is deemed invalid." The offer does not state who would judge the evidence, but of course the judges would be appointed by the antis themselves. If a suit were to be filed to collect the reward, the court might rule that the offer was a gambling bet which should not be enforced by a court. Such a suit would require at least $25,000 for the bond and legal fees. Even if it were won, however, there is no assurance that the money could be recovered from the individuals who sponsor the reward. Most of them are elderly and scattered widely throughout the United States and Canada.

Since the scientific community is so solidly in favor of fluoridation, antis try to discredit it entirely by use of the *conspiracy gambit* (see Chapter 8). The beauty of the conspiracy charge is that it can be leveled at anyone and there is absolutely no way to disprove it. After all, how does one prove that something is not taking place secretly? Favorite "conspirators" are the U.S. Public Health Service, the American Dental Association, the American Medical Association, the Communist Party and the aluminum industry. Apparently, in the minds of the antis, these groups could all be working together to "poison" the American people!

Local promoters are often accused of being in the employ of "vested interests." An individual is rarely accused directly since that could trigger a lawsuit for defamation of character. Instead, a question is asked: "Could it be that Dr. So-and-so is really working for the aluminum industry?" Years ago, the conspiracy gambit would work primarily with the very paranoid. But in the post-Watergate era, it may seem realistic to a wider audience.

"This is only the beginning!" is a related gambit. "First *they* will add fluoride, then vitamin pills, and the next thing you know it will be birth control pills!" Who *"they"* are does not need to be specified.

Scare words will add zip to any anti campaign. Not only the more obvious ones like "cancer" and "heart disease," but also more specialized ones like "mongoloid births" and "sickle cell anemia." *Ecology words* are currently in vogue. Calling fluoride a "chemical" can strike fear in the minds of many Americans who fear we are already too "chemicalized." The fact that water itself is a chemical and the fact that chemists will be sensible and selective will not reassure everyone. Fluoride is called "artificial" and "a pollutant" which is "against nature." Faced with the fact that fluoridation merely copies a natural phenomenon, the antis reply that "natural" fluoride differs from "ar-

168

tificial" fluoride—a fact as yet undiscovered by scientists.

The "against nature" concept led to an exchange which was reported in the Lincoln, Nebraska *Star*. During the fluoridation bill debate, Nebraska State Senator Richard Proud suggested that God would have fluoridated water if he wanted it so treated. Senator Ernest Chambers answered, "And if He had wanted you to smoke, He'd have put a chimney on your head."

Once fluoridation has begun in a community, antis can resort to the *"cause of all evil" gambit*—blaming fluoridation for everything that occurred after it started. An example of this tactic, one that backfired on opponents, took place in Cleveland on June 1, 1956. That was the day fluorides were to be added to the city's water supply. That day, the phone calls began—"My goldfish have died."—"My African violets are wilting."—"I can't make a decent cup of coffee."—"My dog is constipated." Although reactions like this would usually be recognized as psychological, this time their nature was beyond question. Last minute problems had delayed the start of fluoridation for a month!

"Let the People Decide"

The antis' most persuasive argument, both to legislators and to the public, is to call for a public vote. On the surface, this appears to be the democratic way to settle the issue. But the antis are dealing from a stacked deck. First, the people who need fluoridation the most—the children—do not vote. Second, it is not difficult to confuse voters by flooding their community with scare propaganda. The average citizen does not have the educational background to sort out claim and counterclaim or to judge which "authorities" to believe. To turn against fluoridation, he does not need to accept *all* the anti arguments—*just one*. The sheer

169

© King Features Syndicate, Inc., 1973. World rights reserved.

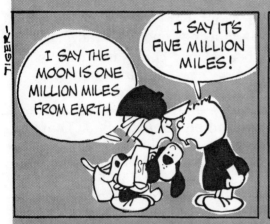

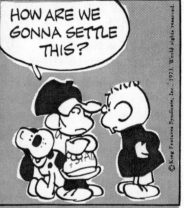

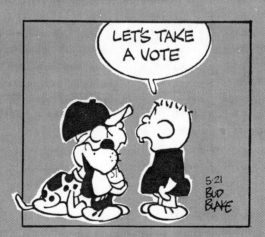

bulk of the controversy is itself likely to arouse doubt in the minds of most voters.

Occasionally, a brave profluoridation group will attempt a referendum as a last resort to overcome the resistance of its local government. But make no mistake about it—the referendum is *primarily* an antifluoridation device. Antis who say, "Let the people decide," may sound as if they wish to use a democratic process to make the decision. But experience in many cities has shown otherwise. If fluoridation wins a referendum, the usual anti response is to work for another one. In a few states where local laws allow repeated referenda on the same subject, fluoridation has been in and out, and in and out again. When this happens, not only do children suffer unnecessary dental costs, but their tax-paying parents pay the high costs of the referenda.

Curiously, studies have shown that referenda can lose even in communities where public opinion favors fluoridation. People will usually go to the polls to vote against whatever they *don't* like. So the crucial factor in many referenda is the ability of proponents to mobilize their supporters.

The value of getting out the vote was never more strikingly demonstrated than in the 1973 referendum in Seattle, Washington. The vote was 115,000 for fluoridation and 49,000 opposed. The key to victory was an unprecedented move by Sheldon Rovin, D.D.S., Dean of the University of Washington School of Dentistry. Two weeks before the election, Dr. Rovin excused students and faculty members from class so that they could participate in a door-to-door campaign. In all, 500 doorbellers saturated the city with their pleas to residents. Person-to-person contact just before the vote worked in Seattle just as it might for any political candidate anywhere—by instructing voters on how to cast their ballots and by giving them a brief opportunity to share their concerns. One homeowner agreed to vote for fluoridation if the canvassers would help him move his television set into the basement.

The Seattle fluoridation forces were extremely well-organized and were very sophisticated politically. They had a broad base of support from community organizations such as unions, the PTA and the Chamber of Commerce. But they also had *no sizable opposition!*

The Devout Anti

Most people who power local and national antifluoridation movements see themselves as saviors of their fellow men. Many of them make opposing fluoridation their single great mission in life. Others include fluoridation among a variety of causes related to health. Antifluoridationists are often active against mental health programs, compulsory immunization and animal research.

Most damaging to the cause of fluoridation are the few antis who are physicians, dentists or others who presumably should be able to judge fluoridation on its merits. Some of them are simply misinformed. Others are alienated for reasons unconnected with fluoridation, but take this cause to get back at the scientific community which they feel has "slighted" them.

What makes a devout anti tick? Three prominent psychiatrists suggested an answer in *Psychodynamics of Group Opposition to Public Health Programs,* an article which appeared in 1960 in the *American Journal of Orthopsychiatry.* Some are motivated by factors of personal power, prestige or gain. Some are driven by great anxieties or hostilities, the sources of which are unconscious. Antis commonly perceive certain health measures as a threat to their "sense of wholeness," and must passionately defend themselves against the "for-

172

cible entry" of any "foreign body" or "foreign agents"—whether this be a vaccination, an interracial contact or a wave of immigrants from overseas. Any of these is apt to be felt as a threat to their "whole way of life."

It is important to realize that a devout anti cannot be dissuaded by facts.

NHF's Cancer Scare

The most active anti in America today is John Yiamouyiannis, Ph.D., "Science Director" of the National Health Federation. Yiamouyiannis is a biochemist who was hired by NHF on June 1, 1974, for the purpose of opposing fluoridation. Since that time, he has written several reports and has traveled throughout the country to give speeches, testify at hearings and meet with legislators. NHF attributes the defeat of the Los Angeles referendum to his vigorous leadership.

Yiamouyiannis is often accompanied by Dean Burk, Ph.D., another biochemist. Burk is a retired employee of the National Cancer Institute, the highly respected branch of the U.S. Public Health Service which evaluates proposed cancer treatments to see if they work. But in recent years, Burk has been a major promoter of the worthless cancer remedy Laetrile.

Yiamouyiannis and Burk claim that fluoridation causes cancer. But their claim is based upon a *misinterpretation* of certain government statistics. In true anti fashion, they compared cancer death rates in fluoridated and non-fluoridated cities. But they failed to consider various factors in each city (such as industrial pollution) which are known to raise the cancer death rate. When the National Cancer Institute did a *genuine* comparative study, it found *no* link between fluoridation and cancer. Undaunted, Yiamouyiannis and Burk charged NCI with a "cover-up." They were joined in this hoax by Congressman James Delaney, who is an anti of long-standing.

Curiously, the National Health Federation has itself been concealing information about fluoridation. In 1972, NHF granted $16,000 for a study to the Center for Science in the Public Interest, a group founded by former associates of Ralph Nader. While it was under way, NHF proudly announced that the study would "put the fluoride controversy into proper perspective." When the study came out *favorable* to fluoridation, however, NHF suddenly became silent about it (see Chapter 13).

Don't Be Misled

As a public health measure, fluoridation is unusual in several ways. It is a copy of a naturally occurring phenomenon. It is supported by libraries full of articles which document its safety and effectiveness—more so than any other public health measure. It is supported by a variety of health, scientific and other civic groups which could hardly be expected to agree on any other single measure. But most significant, it is the only health measure which is often put to public vote.

If you live in a community with fluoridated water, consider yourself lucky. If you do not, don't let the poisonmongers scare you. Fluoridation is a modern health "miracle."

12

THE CONFUSED CRUSADERS

They are everywhere.

BY

GILDA KNIGHT
Executive Assistant
American Institute of Nutrition

To believers, they are prophets. To skeptics, they are profiteers. They are everywhere: Adelle Davis' books, Rodale's magazines, Carlton Fredericks' books and TV appearances, Shute's vitamin E claims, Cheraskin's new hope for incurable diseases. And who hasn't heard about Linus Pauling?

The High Priestess

Adelle Davis used to say that she never saw anyone get cancer who drank a quart of milk daily (as she did). In May 1974, she died of cancer. But behind her she left a trail of ten million books sold and a large and devoted public following.

Ms. Davis promoted hundreds of nutritional tid-bits and theories, many of which were unfounded. She stated incorrectly that fertile eggs were better than infertile eggs, and that crib deaths could be prevented by breast feeding plus vitamin E. Most of her ideas were harmless unless carried to extremes, but some were very dangerous. She opposed pasteurization of milk. She suggested magnesium as a treatment for epilepsy. And she recommended dangerously high doses of vitamins A and D.

In 1971, a four-year old victim of Adelle Davis' advice was hospitalized at the University of California Medical Center in San Francisco. The child appeared pale and chronically ill. She had been having diarrhea, vomiting, fever and loss of hair. Her liver and spleen were enlarged and other physical signs suggested she had a brain tumor. Her mother, "a food faddist who read Adelle Davis religiously," had been giving her large doses of vitamins A and D plus calcium lactate. Fortunately, when these supplements were stopped, the little girl's condition improved.

Adelle Davis was almost the only "health authority" among modern food faddists who possessed any formal professional background. She was trained in dietetics

176

and nutrition at the University of California at Berkeley, and got an M.S. degree in biochemistry from the University of Southern California in 1938. Many of her former classmates and teachers have affectionate memories of her past promise and were greatly distressed about her subsequent activities. Her books, which are full of inaccuracies, are not on the approved list of any bona fide nutrition society.

Let's Eat Right to Keep Fit was Ms. Davis' most popular book. Professor George Mann of the Vanderbilt University School of Medicine found that this book averaged one mistake per page and that some of its errors are actually dangerous. One is the suggestion that certain patients with kidney disease should take potassium chloride—a treatment that could prove fatal.

In *Let's Get Well,* Ms. Davis listed 2,402 references to "document" its 34 chapters. Readers may be impressed with this enormous list, but investigators find that the references often do not back up what she says in the book. In Chapter 12, for example, 27 of 57 listed references contain no data to support her. A reference given in her discussion of "lip problems" and vitamins turns out to be an article about influenza, apoplexy and aviation, with mention of neither lips nor vitamins.

In April, 1972, a group of distinguished nutritionists had the opportunity to ask Adelle Davis what scientific evidence backed up many of her theories. But, like most food faddists, she did not base her ideas on such evidence. To question after question she answered, "I will accept your criticism," "I could be wrong," or "I'm not saying it always does." And she did not modify what she told her followers.

The Consultant

In contrast to Adelle Davis, Carlton Fredericks has had virtually no nutritional or health science training.

He graduated from the University of Alabama in 1931 with a major in English and a minor in political science. His only science courses were two hours of physiology and eight hours of elementary chemistry. He had various jobs until 1937 when he began to write advertising copy for the U.S. Vitamin Corporation and to give sales talks, adopting the title of "nutrition educator."

Records of the City Magistrates' Court of New York show that Fredericks began diagnosing patients and prescribing vitamins for their illnesses. After investigation by agents of the New York State Department of Education, Fredericks was charged with practicing medicine without a license. In April 1945, after pleading guilty, he paid a fine of $500.

In 1955, Fredericks received his Ph.D., having taken no courses in nutrition at all. His thesis topic was *A Study of the Responses of a Group of Adult Female Listeners to a Series of Educational Radio Programs* (his own radio programs).

The Recommended Dietary Allowance of vitamin A is 5,000 international units. Fredericks has advocated daily use of up to 100,000 units for acne and 150,000 to 200,000 for bronchial asthma. Not only are such doses expensive, but they can produce severe nervous system damage.

Fredericks is one of the originators of the crusade to discredit sugar. He has deftly channeled this single theme into a number of variations which reflect and exploit current public concerns about alcoholism, mental disorders and hypoglycemia (low blood sugar). When introduced on the Merv Griffin show as a "leading nutritional consultant," Fredericks was asked to estimate the number of Americans suffering from hypoglycemia. His reply was "20 million." This grossly absurd statement has no basis in fact. Hypoglycemia is very rare. A few years ago, each of the past-presidents of the American Diabetes Association was asked to estimate how many patients he has seen with disorders of blood sugar. All replies were similar: thousands of patients with diabetes (high blood sugar), but *almost none* with functional hypoglycemia.

Carlton Fredericks is a persuasive man with a charming manner. He uses humor to illustrate his points and to ridicule licensed physicians. He encourages self-treatment this way, and encourages self-diagnosis with his scare techniques.

The Chemist

Throughout his most widely known book, *Vitamin C and the Common Cold,* Linus Pauling is convinced that large doses of vitamin C can prevent colds and decrease their severity. Pauling states that daily intake of 200 milligrams (mg.) will decrease the incidence of colds by about 15% and that daily intake of 1,000 mg. will decrease colds by 45%. (The Recommended Dietary Allowance of vitamin C is 40 mg.) Pauling bases his beliefs upon his readings of experiments done by others plus his own personal experience. Looking at the same data, however, the majority of nutrition experts take issue with him.

Scientific fact is established when the same experiment is carried out over and over with the same results. To test the effect of vitamin C on colds, it is necessary to compare groups which get the vitamin to similar groups which get a placebo (a dummy pill which looks like the real thing). Since the common cold is a very variable illness, proper tests must involve hundreds of people for significantly long periods of time.

In 1972, Dr. Terence W. Anderson of the University of Toronto School of Hygiene published the results of a study designed to test Pauling's idea that 1,000 mg. daily would reduce colds by 45%. The incidence of colds was not significantly reduced. However, the group which took the vitamin spent 30% fewer days at home because of illness. To further explore that finding, Dr. Anderson conducted two more experiments in which volunteers took various dosages. Again, vitamin C did not appear to prevent colds or reduce the length of illness. It did appear to reduce the severity of the symptoms—but this could be accomplished with dosages considerably less than those advocated by Pauling. The Anderson experiments have not been confirmed by others. More work is needed to determine whether vitamin C is of practical value in the symptomatic treatment of the common cold.

Pauling has also recommended massive doses of vitamins for the treatment of severe mental illness. The vast majority of psychiatrists and nutritionists do not support this idea, and a recent American Psychiatric Association task force which reviewed the evidence found it entirely lacking.

Curiously, in a little-publicized chapter in his book, Pauling attacks the health food industry for misleading its customers. Pointing out that "synthetic" vitamin C is identical with "natural" vitamin C, he warns that the higher priced "natural" products are a "waste of money." And he adds that "The words 'organically grown' are essentially meaningless—just part of the jargon used by health food promoters in making their excess profits, often from elderly people with low incomes."

Despite these criticisms, Pauling has been welcomed with open arms by the health food industry. His megavitamin views may not be accepted by scientists, but they have been accepted by a large segment of the public. After all, he's a distinguished Nobel Prize winner. That's good enough for John Q. Public, who does not know that Pauling is not a nutritionist.

The Dentist

Like Linus Pauling, Emanuel Cheraskin is a professional who is trained in one area but professes expertise in quite another. A dentist, he has been promoting a wide variety of questionable nutritional ideas in papers for professionals and books for the general public.

In *New Hope for Incurable Diseases,* Dr. Cheraskin and his co-author W. M. Ringsdorf, Jr., another dentist, make many wild claims. Thiamin in 2 mg. doses will increase intelligence up to five times. Vitamin C will improve the behavior of schizophrenics. Carrot and lettuce juice make the hair shine. Liver juice helps diabetics, and spinach juice gives an extra boost of energy. The book makes recommendations which can be cruelly disappointing, if not actually dangerous. It advocates treatment of glaucoma with vitamin C and promises recovery of 75% of schizophrenics treated with long-term megavitamin therapy. Even harmless advice may be given for a senseless reason. For example: "Eat fresh fruits and vegetables to slow down aging."

In *Psychodietetics,* a later book by Cheraskin, Ringsdorf, and Arline Brecher, the authors maintain that "deteriorating eating habits share a major responsibility" in the rise of violence in our population today. Many of the "documented" statements in this book would not withstand scientific scrutiny. References from questionable sources are quoted alongside those recognized as reliable by the scientific community. An example of what the authors consider to be an important scientific study is that of a biochemist who was attempting to evaluate a children's cereal from a nutrition standpoint. He emulsified both the box and the

181

cereal individually, and then fed *one* white rat the box emulsion and another the cereal. Though experiments in rats do not necessarily apply to humans, the authors find it significant that the rat who ate the box thrived!

The Clinicians

So far we have looked at the theories of people which are based on their review of other people's work. The Shute brothers, however, are physicians in the business of treating patients and publishing their findings. Their primary interest is in vitamin E.

Since vitamin E was synthesized in 1938, physicians as well as laymen have tried using it for many different ailments. In 1946, worldwide interest was aroused by a report from Drs. Evan Shute (an obstetrician and gynecologist), Wilfred Shute (a heart specialist), and Albert Vogelsang. The three doctors claimed that large doses of vitamin E were beneficial in the four major types of heart disease. But these claims could not be confirmed by other groups throughout the world.

In his book, *The Heart and Vitamin E and Related Matters,* Evan Shute recommends vitamin E for the prevention and treatment of high blood pressure, gangrene, nephritis, angina pectoris, varicose veins and other conditions. He also claims it can heal wounds without scars and can prevent senility and stroke if taken daily from an early age.

Evan Shute is Medical Director of the Shute Institute in London, Ontario, which in turn is managed by the Shute Foundation for Medical Research. The Institute is supported by fees and gifts for which the Foundation can issue a tax exempt receipt. In 1949, the Institute began publication of *The Summary,* its "scientific journal." The prime reason for publication of *The Summary,* admits Evan Shute, "was the inability of the Shute Foundation to get its presentations published in North American medical journals." Now that should tell us something! Reputable scientific journals accept only papers in which warranted conclusions are drawn from well-designed experiments—such as those which compare treated and untreated groups. Evan Shute's ideas are *not* based on such studies. In fact, he regards them as "unethical, immoral and illegal!"

Some people believe that vitamin E can turn young and old into bedroom superstars. This myth is based on *animal* experiments in which the vitamin was helpful in treating infertility. But no parallel value has been found in human experiments.

Vitamin E has been described as a vitamin in search of a disease to cure. Its main role today is that of a money maker for vitamin merchants. Some day, perhaps, a better use for vitamin E will be discovered.

The Salesmen

"Man has been a creature of fallacy ever since time began. It seems to be inherent in his make-up to believe in false things. . . In the field of medicine, especially, man seems to delight in being completely taken in." J. I. Rodale, who wrote this in 1954, seemed to understand how gullible people can be. He died in 1972, leaving a publishing empire to his son Robert.

Rodale was a shrewd businessman. His financial success attracted considerable attention in the early 1970's, and the publicity he received boosted his profits even more. By 1975, Rodale Press had an estimated gross income of $25 million per year. *Prevention*, its major magazine, had a circulation of one and one-half million. *Organic Gardening and Farming*, its number two publication, had a circulation of one million.

J. I. Rodale was best known for his interests in "organic farming" and "health foods." Most media accounts of his work regarded him as eccentric, but harmless. A few brief mentions of the unscientific nature of his health concepts appeared in AMA publications, but for the most part he was ignored by medical scientists. In a way, that was unfortunate, because he did a great deal of harm.

Prevention magazine contains easy-to-read articles on a variety of health topics. A few articles contain practical health tips, but most articles are misleading. *Prevention's* overall message is that everyone should supplement his diet with extra nutrients. To support this point of view, the magazine uses most of the sales tactics described by Dr. Herbert in Chapter 8. Articles and editorials give equal weight to valid and invalid research, good and poor reasoning, scientific fact and health nonsense. Readers are told that our food supply is depleted of nourishment. News of nutritional "discoveries" is slanted to suggest that readers who take food supplements are likely to benefit from discoveries which are just around the corner.

A typical issue of *Prevention* carries 60–80 pages of food supplement advertising which costs about $6,000 per page. With rare exception, the ads make no health claims—and this is not accidental. If claims of the type found in the articles and editorials surrounding the ads were placed *in* the ads, sellers could be prosecuted for fraud or misbranding. False claims in the magazine's text, however, are shielded by freedom of the press.

In England, where the law is not as strict, J. I. Rodale, Ltd., markets Natrodale brand food supplements with false claims. Among them: *"Eating bone meal will prevent insect bites, will almost completely stop cavities and will lower the pulse when it is high,"* and *"Desiccated liver enormously increases energy."*

Rodale's ideas are summarized into the "Prevention System for Better Health," a mixture of sense and nonsense. Its sensible ideas include avoiding smoking and coffee, and getting proper exercise and nutrition. What is in error, however, is its recommendation of large amounts of supplementary nutrients which are a waste of money. *Prevention's* warnings against sugar, white bread, roast beef, pickles, ice cream, bagels and many other common foods are silly, but relatively harmless. Sugar is accused of "causing criminals," and bread is blamed for colds, rickets in children, steatorrhea in adults, stomach irritation, bronchitis, pneumonia and conjunctivitis. And so on.

Some people who laugh at Rodale Press's silliness may think of its overall set-up as harmless. After all, they say, Rodale does encourage people to do things which may improve their health. But nutritional scientists who look closely at Rodale Press are not amused. Its publications are a significant factor in the growing public confusion about nutrition. And its political activities can cause a great deal of harm.

Although water fluoridation is an extremely valuable way to prevent tooth decay, Rodale opposition to water fluoridation has been very vigorous. Before the death of J. I. Rodale, most issues of *Prevention* contained antifluoridation articles, editorials or letters-to-the-editor. It seems likely that over the years, many rural Americans have become needlessly frightened about fluoridation as a direct result of Rodale misinformation. Communities around Rodale's headquarters in Emmaus, Pa., have been subject to a steady stream of antifluoridation propaganda. In 1961, for example, Rodale Press spent more than $10,000 on a scare campaign which defeated a fluoridation referendum in nearby Allentown.

Rodale Press promotes bone meal tablets as a tooth decay preventive even though scientific authorities know that they are not effective. In 1971, the Lehigh Valley Committee Against Health Fraud published an interesting observation. Ads for bone meal tablets occupied more than $50,000 worth of advertising space in *Prevention* during 1970. In addition, advertisements for filters which were claimed to remove fluorides occupied many additional thousands of dollars of space.

Scientists are also disturbed by Rodale's unfair criticism of pesticides and agricultural chemicals which are badly needed to prevent starvation in many parts of the world (see Chapter 9).

In late 1971, Robert Rodale began a syndicated newspaper column called *Organic Living* which promoted romantic ideas about "nature" with only an occasional hint that our diets are deficient. To promote use of the column, *Prevention* readers were urged to contact local newspaper editors. After a year, some forty newspapers were using Rodale's column, but editorial interest did not last. "Editors stopped using it," according to a source inside Rodale Press, so Rodale stopped writing it during 1975.

Since the death of J. I. Rodale in 1972, Rodale Press has been trying hard to improve its image. *Prevention* contains fewer of the more ridiculous types of ideas which J. I. used to publish. Its articles are more subtle, with less direct suggestion that vitamins will cause miraculous states of health. Readers are still encouraged to supplement their diets with nutrients, both as part of the Prevention System and by slanted articles. Antifluoridation articles are not being published, although occasional letters-to-the-editor from antifluoridation groups assist the groups to raise funds. Rodale Press has also been trying to increase its status by giving money to colleges. But frequent articles in *Prevention* have urged readers to ask their Congressmen to weaken the FDA's ability to protect consumers against misleading nutritional sales claims (see Chapter 13).

Subtle or not, Rodale Press remains one of the nation's leading promoters of health misinformation. Its readers will spend an estimated $300 million for vitamins, minerals and food supplements this year because they believe in Rodale's mythology. But the children who get toothaches or empty bellies—as a result of Rodale's efforts against fluoridation and scientific agriculture—will not understand the source of their suffering.

Recommended Reading

The Vitamin Conspiracy, by John J. Fried, published by E. P. Dutton & Co., New York.

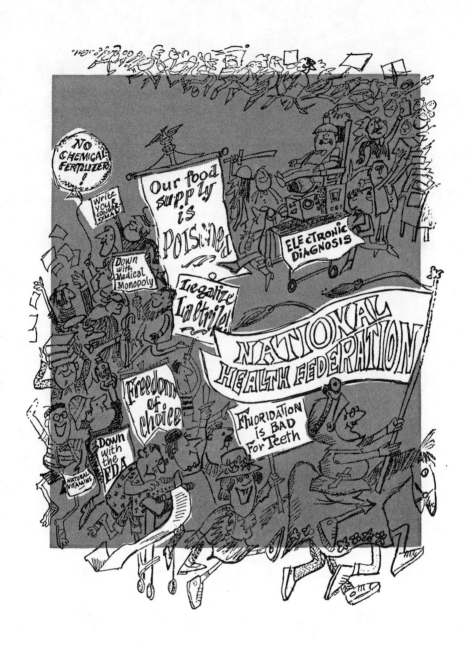

13

THE UNHEALTHY ALLIANCE

Promoters, fighting for the right to cheat.
Victims, fighting for the right to be cheated.

BY

STEPHEN BARRETT, M.D.
Chairman, Board of Directors
Lehigh Valley Committee Against Health Fraud, Inc.

During the past four years, Congress has been flooded with mail urging it to *weaken* government protection in the field of health. Responding to this pressure, most Congressmen became sponsors of legislation which would do exactly that. This strange situation was the result of an intense campaign led by an organization called the National Health Federation (NHF).

Millions of Americans waste money on vitamins, minerals and other "food supplements" which they do not need. Some buyers fear that the American food supply cannot give them enough nourishment. Others hope that nutritional "gimmicks" are the "key" to superior health. About four years ago, after ten years of study, the U.S. Food and Drug Administration (FDA) proposed a number of marketing rules to combat this public confusion. Under these rules, many misleading tactics commonly used by "health food" marketers would be forbidden.

NHF responded immediately with an all-out campaign to weaken the FDA. Lawsuits were filed to block the new FDA rules and Congress was urged to lessen FDA jurisdiction over food supplements and the claims which help to sell them.

NHF's Leaders

The reason for NHF involvement in this issue is suggested by the backgrounds of its leaders. Many of them write or publish books and other materials which support unscientific health theories and practices. Many sell questionable "health" products and some have even been convicted of crimes while engaged in this kind of activity.

• Fred J. Hart, NHF's founder, was for many years the president of the Electronic Medical Foundation. In 1954, Hart and the Electronic Medical Foundation were ordered by a U.S. District Court to stop distributing 13 electrical devices with false claims that they could diagnose and treat hundreds of diseases and conditions. In 1962, Hart was fined by the court for violating this order. Hart died in 1975.

• Royal S. Lee, a non-practicing dentist who died in 1967, helped Hart found NHF and served on its board of governors. In 1962, he and the vitamin company which he owned were convicted of misbranding 115 special dietary products by making false label claims for the treatment of more than 500 diseases and conditions. Lee received a one-year suspended prison term and his company was fined $7,000.

• Andrew G. Rosenberger, a "nature" food store operator, has been listed as NHF "nutrition chairman" and has been a featured speaker at NHF conventions. In 1962, he and his brother Henry were fined $5,000 each and were given six-month suspended prison sentences for misbranding dietary products. Their corporation, Nature Food Centers, was fined $10,000.

• Kurt W. Donsbach, chairman of NHF's board of governors, is a chiropractor and naturopath by background. In 1970, while Donsbach operated a "health food" store, agents of the Fraud Division of the California Bureau of Food and Drug observed him represent that vitamins, minerals and herbal tea would control cancer, cure emphysema and the like. Charged with nine counts of such illegal activity, Donsbach pleaded guilty to practicing medicine without a license and agreed to cease "nutritional consultation." Most of the products which Donsbach was "prescribing" to his "patients" were packaged by a company which he operated at that time. At present, Donsbach is president of Metabolic Products, a company which "specializes in orthomolecular concepts." Literature from Metabolic Products suggests that its garlic extract can

191

"prevent cellular deterioration," that its alfalfa product has "anti-toxin properties" which can help to overcome "-itis" diseases, and so on.

• V. Earl Irons, vice-chairman of NHF's board of governors, received a one-year prison sentence in 1957 for misbranding "Vit-Ra-Tox," a vitamin mixture sold door-to-door.

• Roy F. Paxton, while serving as an NHF governor in 1963, was sentenced to three years in prison for misbranding "Millrue" as effective in treating cancer, arthritis and other serious diseases. One way Millrue was sold was by mail through ads in an NHF publication.

• Clinton Miller, vice-president and Washington lobbyist, had a quantity of "dried Swiss whey" seized from his Utah wheat shop in 1962. The FDA charged that the product was misbranded as effective in treating intestinal disorders. The whey was returned when Miller agreed to change its labeling. In 1976, NHF announced that Miller was a candidate for the United States Senate.

• Bruce Helvie, an NHF governor, had vitamin and mineral products seized by the FDA because they were marketed with false and misleading claims for treatment of more than 25 diseases and conditions. The seized products were destroyed by consent decree in 1960.

• Bob Hoffman, another governor, owns a publishing firm and sells "health" products through his company, York Barbell Co. In 1960, the company was charged with misbranding its "Energol Germ Oil Concentrate" because literature which accompanied the oil claimed falsely that it could prevent or treat more than 120 diseases and conditions, including epilepsy, gallstones and arthritis. The material was destroyed by consent decree. In 1961, fifteen other York Barbell products were seized as misbranded. In 1968, a larger number of products came under attack by the government for similar reasons. In the consent decree which settled the 1968 case, Hoffman and York Barbell agreed to stop a long list of unproven health claims for their products. In 1972, the FDA seized a shipment of three types of York Barbell protein supplements, charging that they were misbranded with false and misleading body-building claims. A few months later, the seized products were destroyed under a default decree.

• Emory Thurston, another NHF governor, has been an active promoter of "Laetrile," a worthless cancer "remedy." Pro-Laetrile pamphlets edited by him were displayed at his booth at an NHF convention at Anaheim, California, in 1973. When approached by an agent of the California Bureau of Food and Drug, who told him she had cancer of the uterus, Thurston said he could supply her with Laetrile. He instructed the agent to contact him at his office at the Institute for Nutritional Research in Hollywood. She did. During their next meeting, Thurston sold Laetrile to the agent—*and advised her not to have surgery!* After additional evidence against Thurston was gathered, he was convicted, fined $500 and placed on probation for two years.

Others who now serve, or who have recently served, on the 27-man NHF board of governors include:

• Harald J. Taub, editor of *Let's Live,* a magazine whose articles strongly promote the use of food supplements. Taub is a former editor of Rodale Press' *Prevention* magazine (see Chapter 12).

• John Hemauer, past-president of the California Chiropractic Association.

• John W. Noble, past-president of the National Association of Naturopathic Physicians, who died in 1976.

• L. P. DeWolf, who, according to NHF, has had "40 years of experience in the organic produce field."

• Betty Lee Morales, president of the Cancer Control Society, a group which promotes unproven cancer "remedies" (see Chapter 1). She is also a publisher and a co-owner of Eden Ranch, a firm which sells *Betty Lee Morales Signature Brand* food supplements. Promotional material from Eden Ranch suggests that Americans who do not use food supplements run a significant risk of developing deficiency diseases.

How NHF Is Organized

The National Health Federation is a membership organization with headquarters in Monrovia, California, and a legislative office in Washington, D.C. Its members pay from $8 per year for "regular" membership to a total sum of $1,000 or more for "perpetual" membership. Many of the larger donors have financial interests in the matters promoted by NHF.

Because of the extent of its political activities, NHF could not qualify as a charitable organization so that contributions to it would be deductible for federal income tax purposes. However, NHF advertisements and letters of welcome to new members have stated otherwise. In 1972, responding to a complaint from the Lehigh Valley Committee Against Health Fraud, Inc., the Internal Revenue Service ordered NHF to stop misrepresenting its tax status.

NHF members receive a monthly 32-page *Bulletin* and occasional brief mailings. They are also invited to frequent conventions, most of which take place in the Western part of the U.S. Visitors to such meetings have noted that most of their participants are persons of middle-age or older who are preoccupied with their health. Many exhibit a rigidly suspicious outlook, fearing that government is thoroughly failing to protect them from "poisons" in their food and from exploitation by medical and drug industries. In November 1974, during a brief visit to an NHF convention in New York City, I noted that at least five of its 34 exhibitors were making misleading sales claims for their products. Most blatant was the claim that a sea-water concentrate would prevent cancer.

According to the *National Health Federation Handbook*, available for ten cents, any two members can start a local chapter by adopting the NHF constitution and bylaws, naming temporary officers and receiving clearance from NHF headquarters. The *Handbook* envisions a pyramidal national structure with local groups selecting a county board of directors, county boards selecting a state board of governors and state boards selecting one delegate each to join 21 at-large governors at the national level. This structure is mainly hypothetical, however, since the number of local chapters is too small. (An article in the July 1972 *Bulletin* reported the formation of NHF's 85th local chapter.) National membership, estimated from *Bulletin* circulation figures was about 24,000 in 1973, 20,750 in 1974 and 18,500 in 1975. NHF's budget was reported to be $345,000 in both 1975 and 1976.

NHF's Philosophy

Since its formation in 1955, the steadfast purpose of NHF has been to promote what it calls "freedom of choice" by health consumers. As stated in each issue of its monthly *Bulletin:*

> "NHF opposes monopoly and compulsion in things related to health where the safety and welfare of others are not concerned. NHF does not oppose nor approve any specific healing profession or their methods, but it does oppose

the efforts of any one group to restrict the freedom of practice of qualified members of another profession, thus attempting to create a monopoly."

At first glance, this credo may seem harmless and somehow related to opposing unfair business competition. What NHF really means, however, is that scientific methods of treatment should not be allowed to drive quackery out of the marketplace. Under this philosophy, anyone who has a product or a "treatment" which he claims can help sick people should be allowed to sell it. Proof that a particular method works should not be required. People should be free to decide for themselves which health care measures they will use. Unless a method causes immediate death or serious injury, our government should not interfere.

Put in its simplest terms, what the National Health Federation wants is for quackery to be made legal.

The Scope of NHF Activity

NHF's publications and convention programs make it clear that NHF promotes the gamut of questionable health methods and has little interest in medically acceptable types of treatment.

Nutritional fads, myths and gimmicks are given favorable mention by NHF *Bulletin* articles, by convention speakers and special mailings and by pamphlets available at conventions and by mail. Worthless cancer treatments such as Laetrile and Krebiozen are promoted in the same ways. *Bulletin* articles look with disfavor upon such proven health measures as pasteurization of milk, smallpox vaccination, polio vaccination and fluoridation of water. Use of nutritional supplements is encouraged by claims that our food processing depletes its nutrients. Use of "natural" products is encouraged by exaggerated claims that our food supply is "poisoned." Chiropractic is regarded favorably. Books which promote questionable health concepts are reviewed favorably in the *Bulletin.* Underlying all these messages is the idea that anyone who opposes NHF ideas is part of a "conspiracy" of government, organized medicine and big business against the little consumer.

NHF files many lawsuits against government agencies and joins in the defense of people accused of frauds in the sale of questionable "health" products. It also has an active legislative program with a Washington-based lobbyist.

NHF was active in support of chiropractic inclusion under Medicare and in opposition to federal subsidies to communities who want fluoridation. To bolster the influence of its lobbyist, the *Bulletin* and special mailings include form letters and instructions to write to Congressmen and Federal officials in support of NHF positions. Letter-writing requests invariably contain misinformation about the issues and contain underlying themes of persecution, discrimination and conspiracy. For example, to arouse support for the anti-FDA vitamin bill, NHF suggested that FDA regulations would drive up prices, "take away our vitamins" and even make it illegal to manufacture most of the supplements now available.

Crying, "Fight for your freedom to take vitamins!," NHF organized its members and allies into unprecedented political activity. Article after article urging support of the anti-FDA bill appeared in the NHF *Bulletin,* in *Prevention* magazine and other health food industry publications, and in chiropractic journals. Letter-writing kits were distributed by chiropractors, health food stores and in special NHF mailings. At a Congressional hearing held on this issue, several Congressmen reported that they received more mail about vitamins than about Watergate! As the mail piled up, most Congressmen lost sight of why it was coming— that their constituents had been confused and frightened by health food industry propaganda. In 1976, a modified form of NHF's anti-FDA bill was passed by Congress.

In 1973, a New Jersey-based group called Citizens for Truth in Nutrition (CTN) was formed. Although apparently independent from NHF, it was led by many NHF activists. Its major activities included anti-FDA meetings, media appearances and anti-FDA lawsuits. Like NHF, CTN's promotional literature claimed falsely that its contributions were tax-deductible until it was ordered to stop these claims by the Internal Revenue Service.

NHF's Fight Against Fluoridation

Scientists know that if children get the proper amount of fluoride in their diet, they will get many fewer cavities in their teeth. Adjusting community drinking water to about one part fluoride to one million parts water is a safe and simple way to accomplish this. Although NHF's leaders claim to be interested in preventing disease by "proper" nutrition, they fight hard against water fluoridation.

Over the years, NHF has assembled a great many "documents" which it claims are "proof" that fluoridation is dangerous (which it is not). Close examination of these documents, however, shows that they contain reports of poorly designed "experiments," twisted accounts of actual events, statements by respected scientists taken out of context to change their meaning, misinterpreted statistics and other forms of faulty reasoning. Given enough publicity, however, these items can convince many communities that fluoridation is too risky. Many innocent American children have NHF to thank for their toothaches.

In January 1972, NHF granted $16,000 for a fluoridation study to the Center for Science in the Public Interest (CSPI), a group led by former associates of Ralph Nader. To help raise this money, a special mailing was sent to NHF members:

"SPECIAL URGENT APPEAL = NHF is proud to announce that it has undertaken to underwrite $16,000.00 in costs for the CLINICALLY controlled investigation of the long-term effects of fluorides in the human. This test is being conducted by FRIENDS of indisputable, scientific reputation. With this information we will be armed with unassailable, up-to-date, scientific data to help defeat fluoridation! There is NO such study available in the world at this time and the costs are amazingly low. The Executive Committee committed us to this obligation in emergency session. . ."

When CSPI learned about this fund-raising message, it protested, stating that its study would be a scientific review of available knowledge and that the outcome was certainly not fixed against fluoridation. NHF apologized, claiming that the fund-raiser had been mailed "without being cleared by appropriate officials" and contained "serious errors" about the nature of the study.

In August 1972, a preliminary draft of the CSPI study was released to activists on both sides of the fluoridation controversy. This was done so that its author could get suggestions and criticisms from knowledgeable individuals before he wrote his final report. The final report was issued at about the same time as the December 1972 NHF *Bulletin* went to press stating:

199

"A good many months ago, NHF voted a grant to the Center for Science in the Public Interest to underwrite an unbiased study of total fluoride consumption and its influence on health. This was done on the anticipation that such a study, never before undertaken by a scientific body, would put the fluoride controversy into proper perspective. That study is nearing its completion. Two preliminary, interim reports have been issued. It begins to appear as if most of the contentions of NHF on this question will be validated in this unbiased study."

CSPI's final report, however, did not "validate most of NHF's contentions." Rather, it concluded that ". . . the known benefits of fluoridation far outweigh any risks which may be involved."

The study was never again mentioned in NHF publications. In private communications, however, NHF claimed first that the study "was never completed" and later that it was unacceptable because its author ignored too much anti-fluoridation "evidence." A Rodale Press editor suggested that the author had been "intimidated" or "bought off."

Thus, having invested $16,000 in an "unbiased" study by "FRIENDS of indisputable, scientific reputation," NHF ignored its conclusions.

During 1974, NHF announced that opposing fluoridation would be its number two priority and that a biochemist named John Yiamouyiannis had been hired to "break the back" of fluoridation promotion (see Chapter 11).

The Unique Alliance

NHF thus stands revealed. Its policies disregard medical science and proven public health measures. Its leaders promote questionable "health" methods, often at personal profit. Its followers, although confused about the issues in which they involve themselves, are active in the arena of politics.

NHF is well-organized and working hard. Its leaders probably hold sincere beliefs in their health methods. Its followers sincerely believe they can improve their health by following the methods of their leaders.

Sincere or not, however, NHF may be dangerous to your health!

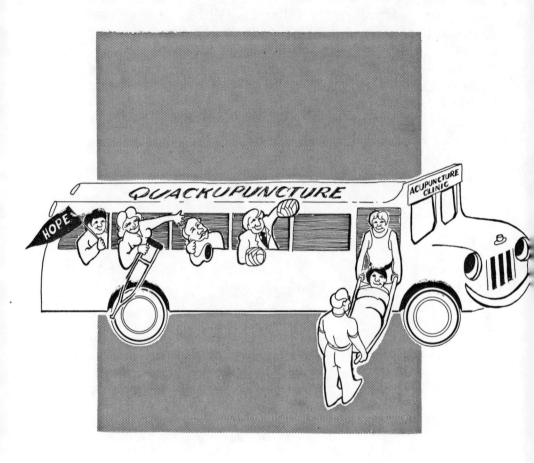

14

QUACKUPUNCTURE?

Q: "Did acupuncture relieve you of your problem?"
A: "No. It just relieved me of my money."

BY

ARTHUR TAUB, M.D., Ph.D.
Professor, Clinical Anesthesiology
Director, Section for the Study and Treatment of Pain
Yale University School of Medicine

Immediately before and after the visit of former President Richard M. Nixon to the People's Republic of China in 1971, reports were circulated in the West by visitors to China suggesting that major surgery could be accomplished with the use of acupuncture alone as the anesthetic agent. The impression was given that acupuncture was widely used, that it could be used in high risk cases, in children, in the aged, and in veterinary surgery. Perhaps the best known rumor about "acupuncture anesthesia" was that the New York Times' journalist, James Reston, had his appendix removed with acupuncture as the anesthetic. Whatever the reasons for these ideas having gained currency, they are, every single one of them, untrue.

Acupuncture As a System of Medicine

Chen-Chiu, or acupuncture-moxibustion, is a technique of medical treatment which began in Stone Age China. It consists of the insertion of needles into the skin, or muscles and tendons beneath, at one or more named points. These points are generally found where imaginary horizontal and vertical lines meet on the surface of the body. These points are said to "represent" various internal organs. The organs are also "represented" by acupuncture points on the surface of the ear or on one finger. Good health is said to be produced by a harmonious mixture of Yin and Yang, the fundamental activity characteristics of the universe, which combine to form the life force, or Ch'i. The disorganization of the flow of Ch'i is said to produce illness. The acupuncture needle supposedly can regulate this flow. Moxibustion is a technique in which the herb *Artemesia Vulgaris*, or wormwood, is burned at specified points on or near the skin, sometimes to the point of blistering.

Classical Chinese physicians applied these tech-

204

niques to the entire range of human illness. Surgery as such (save for the operation of castration used to supply eunuchs for the imperial household) was not a part of classical Chinese medicine. The diagnosis of disease was based mainly upon the diagnosis of the "pulse." This was not a measurement of the rate and rhythm of the heart, as is done nowadays. Rather, the "pulse" was related to such things as the "texture" and force of the radial artery at several points of the wrist, while the artery was being compressed lightly or forcefully. The feeling imparted to the finger of the pulse diagnostician revealed the state of health of the various internal organs. Diagnosis was also based upon the history of the patient's symptoms and on the state of the weather. Because dissection of the human body was not practiced, internal organs were imagined in rather odd positions and shapes. Pseudoviscera, or non-existent organs, were invented. One of these was the so-called "triple warmer," whose precise location baffles the most astute translator of Chinese acupuncture classics.

Herbal pharmacology played and continues to play a significant role in classical Chinese medicine. Herbs were generally made into a sort of tea. Some of these herbs possess useful therapeutic properties (such as the herb Ma Huang, which is known to contain ephedrine, a drug useful in the treatment of asthma). The majority of such preparations, however, are worthless. In recent years, many classical preparations have been "adulterated" with active agents which have not been listed as ingredients.

Classical Chinese medicine was practiced for thousands of years, maintained by the force of Buddhist and Confucian conservatism. Discerning Chinese were not always content with it, however, particularly when other forms of medical and surgical treatment became known to them.

Resistance to Acupuncture in China

In the late 19th century, efforts of the waning Manchu dynasty toward modernization included an unsuccessful attempt to forbid acupuncture. In the following years, vigorous opposition to acupuncture was mounted by both right and left-wing intellectuals. Notable among the latter group was Lu Hsun, today a major figure in the literature of the People's Republic of China, and an author much favored by the late Communist Party Chairman Mao Tse Tung. Lu Hsun ridiculed traditional notions of physiology and indicted Chinese medicine for ineptness, ignorance and greed. These indictments were echoed in the 30's and 40's by Pa Chin, a revolutionary writer. Many conservative Chinese Nationalist intellectuals shared these authors' feelings of revulsion toward acupuncture and Chinese medicine. Repeated attempts by the Kuomintang to forbid acupuncture failed primarily because of political pressure. In spite of its low therapeutic value, many party members saw Chinese medicine as a part of the "national essence." Prior to the military unification of Mainland China in 1948–9, the Chinese Communist Party did not place emphasis upon acupuncture as a major medical technique. In fact, in Communist China today, Norman Bethune, a Canadian surgeon (certainly a non-acupuncturist) who died in action with the 8th Route Army in the war against Japan, is a hallowed figure. His statue appears in almost every major museum and public building. His bravery, dedication, and medical and surgical skill are held up as examples for the Chinese people at large to emulate.

Even though the Chinese Communist Party has made an intensive effort to eliminate traditional modes of thought and to reform social structure, acupuncture has been kept as an integral portion of its national medical system. The Party realized that the approximately 10,000 western-trained physicians in China at the time of the Chinese Communist Revolution were too few to carry out the gigantic public health tasks necessary to modernize China. Medical personnel would therefore have to be recruited from among the approximately 500,000 practitioners of traditional Chinese medicine. It was apparently expected that these practitioners would gradually become more scientific in their work. As Chairman Mao put it, "Traditional Chinese medicine and pharmacology are a great treasure house. Efforts must be made to explore them and raise them to a higher level." The efforts of the Communist Party to elevate traditional Chinese practitioners, however, have been hampered by the Party's other political doctrines. As a result, unscientific medical practices remain widespread throughout China.

Acupuncture Quackery

Claims that acupuncture is effective are publicly advanced without evidence to back them up.

One strategy by which the Chinese maintain this fiction is to use acupuncture therapy simultaneously with known effective medication. For example, a recent Chinese textbook states, "Epilepsy is generally caused by rising air and congestion causing the heart to be stuffed and confused. The disease is in the heart, the liver, and the bladder. Treatment should be designed to ease the liver, to stop the rising air, to eliminate congestion and to open up stuffed circulation." Six kinds of herbal medicine mixtures are then advocated. Three forms of acupuncture are also included. Vitamins are injected into one of the acupuncture points. However, the effective medications diphenylhydantoin, phenobarbital and primidone are also suggested. For myasthenia gravis, a disease in which muscles including those of breathing are easily fatigued, vigorous physical training methods including cold baths (which could be dangerous in this disease) are suggested by this same textbook. Thirteen useful acupuncture points are discussed, with vitamin injections suggested at some of them. Traditional Chinese herbs are suggested as a "tonic" to improve the "air." Again, however, the effective agents neostigmine, physostigmine and ephedrine are also advised. A similar approach is used in the treatment of parkinsonism ("shaking palsy"). Acupuncture, Chinese herbal medicine, and effective medications such as the belladonna alkaloids are prescribed. There is not the slightest evidence to show that the traditional Chinese medical methods improve the modern treatment of these diseases in any way.

Another strategy adopted by the Chinese to maintain the appearance of the success of acupuncture is the illusion of effective therapy having been given. This is done by suppressing knowledge of the natural course of illnesses which improve spontaneously. Acupuncture is then given credit for curing illnesses which would have improved by themselves.

In May 1974, I was a member of the Acupuncture Study Group of the Committee on Scholarly Communication with the People's Republic of China. Our group visited the Acupuncture Research Institute in Peking as well as traditional medical hospitals in the Shanghai region. There I saw this technique in action. One patient received acupuncture treatment beginning two weeks after a stroke. Patients of this type tend to recover spontaneously and gradually. In fact, this patient, who had received acupuncture for six months, recovered no more and no less than one would be expected to recover with no treatment or with a minimum of physical therapy. Several young women I examined had monthly migraine headaches associated with nausea, vomiting, spots before their eyes and sensitivity to bright light. They told me that monthly acupuncture treatment limited their headaches to a duration of several days per month. They apparently did not know that this is the usual state of affairs without treatment.

Another strategy used by the Chinese is to claim benefit from acupuncture where none, in fact, exists. One nearsighted child I saw was given acupuncture treatment before receiving her eyeglasses. I was told that the degree of her optical correction would be less as a result of the acupuncture treatment she had received. This was simply untrue. Other patients with Parkinson's disease, spinal cord damage, and after-effects of head injury were also said to have "improved." My examination detected no improvement. Patients are also said to receive treatment for "nerve deafness." However, properly controlled studies conducted recently in the United States have failed to show that acupuncture can help nerve deafness.

"Acupuncture Anesthesia"

Acupuncture is not widely used in China as an "anesthetic." A reasonable estimate of the total use of "acupuncture anesthesia" is approximately five to ten percent. In our May 1974 visit to China, the Acupuncture Study Group was able to substantiate a number of previous reports that almost all patients operated upon under "acupuncture anesthesia" received other agents in addition. This almost always included phenobarbital (a sedative) and meperidine (a narcotic painkiller) before and during the operation. Local anesthesia was also used liberally. I personally witnessed operations in which local anesthesia was used from beginning to end, but which were never-the-less classified as done under "acupuncture anesthesia."

Quackupuncture?

Sometimes acupuncture needles are inserted not only into the skin but as much as several inches beneath the skin directly into major nerve trunks. These can be stimulated with electric shocks to exhaust their ability to conduct impulses and produce local anesthesia. "Acupuncture anesthesia" is not generally used in children under 12 because of their inability to cooperate. Elderly patients are generally not operated upon with "acupuncture anesthesia" and it is considered "experimental" in animals. (When it is done in animals, they are strapped down tightly to the operating table.) On an occasion which I personally witnessed, the animal, a horse, kicked vigorously during the operative procedure, suggesting that anesthesia was not working. The horse also drank with particular eagerness the water that was offered to it, suggesting that it was in surgical shock.

Acupuncture anesthesia is never used for emergency surgery. It is said to be applicable only to "classical" surgery—operations in which no complications are expected. These operations are performed so as to minimize tissue damage and pulling upon muscles or internal organs. To achieve this end, surgical incisions are made small. This means that the operative field is often poorly exposed, increasing the risk that important structures may be damaged. Proper exploration is usually not possible, wasting the opportunity to detect previously undiagnosed disease such as cancer.

The Chinese state that general anesthesia is always available as a "backup" procedure in case the patient experiences overwhelming pain when "acupuncture anesthesia" is used alone. This means, however, that general anesthesia would be started in the midst of an already hazardous surgical situation. The most dangerous time during anesthesia is when the patient is being put to sleep. This is the time where spasms of the vocal cord or arrest of the heart are most likely to occur. If general anesthesia is delayed until severe pain requires it to be used, these dangers are increased.

Despite these drawbacks, a limited number of major surgical procedures have been performed in China using only small amounts of premedication, little or no local anesthetic and the insertion of acupuncture needles. These surgical procedures which have been witnessed have gone well, but postoperative studies have not been done. Proper studies should not only attempt to describe what has taken place, but must also take into account the fact that Western patients differ from Chinese patients in their reactivity to pain and in cultural attitudes toward surgery. Since good statistical studies are not available from the Chinese, "acupuncture anesthesia" should be considered experimental. Doctors who undertake it, and patients who submit to it, should do so only under carefully controlled conditions in established research programs.

Are you wondering what happened to James Reston? The operation to remove his appendix was done with chemical anesthesia. Acupuncture needles were said to have "relieved" his postoperative pain one hour after they had been used. It seems more likely, however, that the relief resulted from the spontaneous return of normal intestinal function.

Acupuncture "Clinics" and Failed Treatment in the United States

The popularization of acupuncture and its supposed therapeutic results has produced an immense development of acupuncture "clinics" and "centers" throughout the United States. In the District of Columbia alone, more than ten such centers are now in operation. While the majority of these "clinics" or "centers" are "supervised" by licensed physicians, acupuncture

211

is performed in the same manner as it has always been performed. Diagnostic investigations are minimal. Previous diagnoses or misdiagnoses are usually accepted, with therapy prescribed by ancient rule of thumb. The patient is generally abandoned to his own devices if acupuncture does not prove successful after a small number of treatments, generally ten or less. As in classical times (and in modern China), treatment is given for disorders in which symptoms vary with the weather and the disposition of the patient, such as generalized osteoarthritis, or for disorders in which remissions are the rule, such as multiple sclerosis. In a recent taped discussion in which I participated, the director of one American acupuncture clinic maintained that patients previously unable to walk because of multiple sclerosis were able to walk out of his clinic unaided. The gentleman did not indicate how he substantiated the diagnosis. Nor could he state what had prevented the patients from walking, whether their legs were weak, their coordination or balance impaired, and the like. Nor could he state how and to what degree these functions had improved as a result of treatment. It should be clear that if a "paralyzed" patient walks unaided after brief treatment, it is certainly more appropriate to question the diagnosis than to praise the treatment!

Along with the increase in the number of acupuncture clinics and centers (some of which provide direct bus transportation from local shopping centers to their premises), there has been an increased number of patients seen in pain and arthritis clinics for whom acupuncture has failed. Among those I have personally attended were:

(1) A middle-aged gentleman with sexual impotence and suicidal depression. He had been treated with acupuncture needles placed in the thighs and in the

region between the penis and the rectum. Later he required psychiatric treatment.

(2) A middle-aged woman with pain in the upper teeth who was treated with acupuncture stimulation with needles placed between the 2nd and 3rd toes of her foot. She required extensive dental diagnosis and treatment, as well as psychiatric care to compensate for the intense feelings of frustration which followed the failure of treatment.

(3) A middle-aged public relations man who was born with a malformed spinal canal. This gentleman had more pain at the end of treatment than when he began.

(4) Patients with osteoarthritis of the hands who showed minimal relief after the first, but increased pain after the last treatments, and who eventually abandoned them as useless.

(5) Patients with neuralgic pain following shingles which acupuncture did not help.

A characteristic remark of my patients was made by a middle-aged man with back pain who said that acupuncture therapy relieved him only of his money.

Does Acupuncture Relieve Pain?

It is reasonably clear that acupuncture does not cure disease. But, does it relieve pain? My clinical experience with acupunctured patients suggests that if any pain relief is produced by the procedure, it is short-lasting. Formal psychological investigations into this problem have shown conflicting results. In most instances, acupuncture produced no better relief than was produced by a placebo. In other studies, acupuncture did produce some degree of difficulty in distinguishing a previously painful from a non-painful stimulus, but this relief was minimal and short-lasting and was not at all comparable with the degree of relief claimed for conventional acupuncture therapy.

Risks of Acupuncture

Acupuncture has not merely failed to demonstrate significant benefits. It has also, in some instances, been extremely dangerous.

Acupuncture needles are not only inserted into the skin. Needles, up to one foot in length (!), may be inserted deep into the body. Serious harm may result when they penetrate vital structures. In one case of back pain and burning around the mouth and vagina, needles were inserted through the skin of the chest. The lung was penetrated. It collapsed, filling the chest cavity with almost a pint of blood. The patient required two weeks of hospitalization which was complicated by pneumonia.

Death from puncture of the heart has been reported. Other reports mention puncture of the liver, spleen, bladder, kidneys and the pregnant uterus.

Since classical Chinese medical practice does not recognize that germs cause disease, acupuncture needles need not be sterilized. Lack of sterile technique will, of course, cause bacterial infections. In China today, acupuncture needles are stored in alcohol solutions. Since alcohol does not kill the virus which causes infectious hepatitis, contaminated needles can spread this serious infection from patient to patient.

Some acupuncture needles are unusually thin and poorly made. Such needles tend to break. One scientist suffered excruciating pain in an acupuncture experiment when the needle broke off in his foot. An operation was needed to remove the needle.

"Acupuncture anesthesia" may include electrical stimulation of needles placed directly into the sciatic nerve (the main nerve to the leg). If the nerve is stimu-

214

lated for several hours with high frequency current, permanent nerve injury is almost guaranteed. The nerve fibers may burn, the nerve sheath may tear, and bleeding into the nerve may occur.

Stimulation of the so-called Ya-men point is recommended for the treatment of nerve deafness in children. Scientific study has demonstrated that this technique is useless. The Ya-men point is located directly above the most sensitive part of the human nervous system, the junction between the spinal cord and the base of the brain. A needle entering this sensitive area can produce instant paralysis of arms and legs, stoppage of breathing, and death.

Textbooks of acupuncture therapeutics advise acupuncture for some conditions which can lead to death or serious disability if not properly diagnosed and treated. Among these conditions are high fever and whooping cough in children, tender breasts in women and urinary difficulties in men.

While adequate training in medicine or in acupuncture techniques may decrease the incidence of complications, this is no comfort to the victims of these complications.

Acupuncture Teaching

It is safe to say that most people who practice acupuncture are not adequately trained either in acupuncture techniques or in medicine. This is particularly true in the United States. For what it is worth, in China, formal training in acupuncture requires several years. Many American practitioners, however, have merely attended "quickie" courses, some of which lasted only one or two days. Chiropractors are flocking to these courses in large numbers. One chiropractor who travels around the country teaching "quickie" courses was asked how long it would take to learn a

215

working knowledge of acupuncture. He replied, "I can teach you all you have to know in ten minutes."

Acupuncture Licensing

Some states are trying to control acupuncture abuse by licensing practitioners. While this may drive some two-day wonders out of the marketplace, it will not solve the entire problem. First, licensing of acupuncture may make it difficult for some well-trained physicians to study it. Second, some legal approaches will result in patients being channeled into acupuncture "centers" of dubious value.

The mythology of acupuncture has spread rapidly through our country. It will be difficult to control. Our best hope is that with time, education and gradual appreciation of its worthlessness, acupuncture will be resisted by the public. Then it will pass beyond us, as have its sister quackeries: purging, leeching, bleeding, *et cetera.*

15

THE EYE EXORCISORS

Don't throw away your glasses.

BY
JACOB NEVYAS, Ph.D., Sc.D.
Professor Emeritus of Chemistry
Pennsylvania College of Optometry

The mistaken belief that poor eyesight can be cured by special eye exercises has been held by many persons since ancient times. This belief was brought to its highest state of fruition by a one-time reputable physician, William Horatio Bates, M.D., who published a volume in 1920 entitled *The Cure of Imperfect Eyesight by Treatment Without Glasses*. The following account is a summary of the work of Dr. Bates and his many followers as described in a book by the late Dr. Philip Pollack, a prominent optometrist of New York City. Entitled *The Truth About Eye Exercises*, it was published in 1957 and is now out of print.

Pollack's book considers Dr. Bates to have been a sincere individual with an impressive record. He was born in Newark, New Jersey, in 1860, graduated from Cornell University in 1881 and from Columbia University's College of Physicians and Surgeons in 1885. For the next seven years, he practiced in New York City as an ethical physician. He specialized in eye, ear, nose and throat diseases and worked in a number of prominent hospitals. In 1902, however, Dr. Bates fell victim to amnesia and disappeared from view. His wife found him seven weeks later working as a doctor's assistant at the Charing Cross Hospital in London, England. Two days later he vanished again and was missing for eight years, during which time his wife died. In 1910, Dr. Bates was found practicing medicine in Grand Forks, North Dakota, and was persuaded to return to New York, where he resumed practice and married again.

Early in his career, Bates displayed an interest in problems of vision. In 1891 he published an article in a medical journal on the cure of near-sightedness by eye exercises. In his office, he taught patients to stare into the sun and to relax their eyes by covering them with their palms. He soon became obsessed with his peculiar theories of vision.

In 1917, Bates teamed up with Bernarr Macfadden, a

nationally known food faddist who published the magazine *Physical Culture*. Together they offered a course in the Bates System of Eye Exercises for a fee which included a subscription to the magazine. This venture met with considerable success and led many readers to believe in the Bates System. However, the big impact of Bates' work materialized after publication of his book. This book attracted large numbers of charlatans, quacks and gullible followers who then published scores of unscientific books and articles on the subject of vision. Extolling the Bates System, these authors urged readers to "throw away" their glasses. Some of these writers established schools which still flourish today.

Contrary to scientific fact, Bates taught that the dimensions of the eyeball and the state of the crystalline lens have nothing to do with poor eyesight. All defects in vision, he said, are caused by eyestrain and nervous tension. To achieve perfect vision, just relax the eyes completely. Bates warned that eye glasses cause the vision to deteriorate. He also deplored the use of sunglasses. Bates claimed his exercises could correct nearsightedness, far-sightedness, astigmatism and presbyopia (the inability of older people to focus their eyes on nearby objects). They could also cure such diseases as cataracts, eye infections, glaucoma and macular degeneration. His exercises were as follows:

1. *Palming:* This is the principal procedure of the Bates System. The patient must first look intently at a black object, then close his eyes and recall to mind its blackness. This procedure supposedly relaxes the eyes, relieves eyestrain, corrects vision to normal and eliminates pain during surgery.

2. *Shifting:* By shifting his gaze continually from object to object, the patient will improve his vision.

3. *Sun Gazing:* Staring directly into the sun, the patient will benefit from the "warmth of light."

4. *Remembering Blackness:* Presbyopia will be

cured when the patient closes his eyes and recalls the condition of "blackness."

It should be obvious that these exercises cannot influence eyesight disorders as Bates claimed. Near-sightedness, far-sightedness and astigmatism result from inborn and acquired dimensions of the lens and the eyeball. Presbyopia is the result of rigidity of the lens. As for eye diseases, the only thing the exercises can do is delay proper medical or surgical treatment and result in permanent impairment of vision. It should also be noted that all eye doctors caution patients against looking directly into the sun. Such a practice can cause permanent damage to the macula, the most sensitive and important area of the retina.

Dr. Bates died in 1931. His office and teaching practices were taken over very successfully by his wife with the help of Dr. Harold M. Peppard. Mrs. Bates had worked with her husband for a number of years and Dr. Peppard was an ardent advocate of the Bates System. In 1944, he published a book called *Sight Without Glasses*. Many other writers of questionable knowledge followed Bates' path. One of the best known was Gayelord Hauser, popular food faddist and favorite of Hollywood, who in 1932 published *Keener Sight Without Glasses*. By combining eye exercise and diet theories, Hauser could further the sale of his own dietary products.

One convert to the Bates System deserves special notice because he had no financial interest in it. This was the well-known British novelist, Aldous Huxley. In 1942 Huxley wrote *The Art of Seeing,* claiming that he personally had been helped by the System. He had been a patient of Mrs. Margaret Dorst Corbett, who wrote four books on the system. Mrs. Corbett also operated two schools for teaching Bates methods to patients and other practitioners. In 1941 Mrs. Corbett was charged with violating the Medical Practice Act of California for treating eyes without a license. Her defense was that she taught only eye relaxation exercises and did not impinge upon the practice of medicine or optometry. She was acquitted and her acquittal met with a large wave of popular approval. A similar case is that of Miss Clara A. Hackett who operated schools in Los Angeles, San Diego and Seattle. Indicted in New York in 1951, she too was acquitted of practicing medicine and optometry without a license.

Many other authors have reached large audiences with their books on the Bates System. Most prominent among them are Bernarr Macfadden (*Strengthening Your Eyes*, 1924); Cecil S. Price (*The Improvement of Sight*, 1934); and Ralph J. Mac Fayden (*See Without Glasses*, 1948). There has even been a mechanical device on the market known as the "Natural Eye Normalizer" for massaging the eyelids to cure all complaints of vision!

It is difficult to understand the widespread popularity of the Bates System unless one considers that its followers make up what is essentially a cult. Its practitioners are *faith healers* who appeal to the gullible, the neurotic, the highly emotional and the psychosomatic. Even the author Mac Fayden admits that the System's results are 90% "mental."

I know of a near-sighted woman who used to travel from Philadelphia to New York City once a week to see a Bates practitioner. She expected that his treatment would eliminate her need for thick glasses. Each trip cost her a day's wages plus train fare, lunch and the practitioner's fee. For several months an optometrist friend of mine tried to convince her that she was wasting her time and money. He finally persuaded her to ask the practitioner what progress she was making and how long it would take before she could change her glasses. At the same time, the optometrist gave her a sealed envelope to open at the end of her next visit in New York.

Questioned by the woman, the practitioner replied, "I was just about to tell you. We have decided that we can improve you no further. You should return to your optometrist for further care." Opening the envelope, the woman saw that the optometrist had predicted the Bates practitioner's reply almost word for word! She finally saw the light.

There is one *rational* method of eye training and eye exercises which must not be confused with the system of Bates and his followers. This is called "Orthoptics." It is used to correct "crossed eyes" and amblyopic or "lazy" eyes. Crossed eyes are caused by an imbalance of the muscles which control eye movements. This condition can often be improved by orthoptics or surgery or a combination of the two. If muscles are out of balance, the function of one eye may become suppressed to avoid double vision. The suppressed eye is known as an "amblyopic" eye. Covering the good eye can often stimulate the amblyopic eye to work again to provide binocular vision for the patient.

Remember—no type of eye exercise can improve refractive errors or cure any diseased conditions within the eye itself.

16

THE GADGETEERS

The miracles of science have made it easy to believe in science fiction.

BY
WALLACE F. JANSSEN
Historian
U.S. Food and Drug Administration

There was dead silence in the courtroom.

The tense little man in the witness chair leaned forward and shook his finger at the jury.

"I had fits all my life till Dr. Ghadiali cured me!" he shouted. *"His Spectrochrome stopped my fits and now I feel grand!"*

Suddenly the witness paled, stiffened in his chair and frothed at the mouth. As he began to convulse, a government physician and courtroom attendants stepped forward, placed something in his mouth and carried him away.

This shocking moment was but one of the dramatic episodes which marked the trial of Dinshah P. Ghadiali, "seventh son of a seventh son," and organizer of a nationwide healing cult which became a religion to his followers.

Ghadiali was a "gadget quack," inventor of the "Spectrochrome," a machine which resembled a theatrical spotlight. Spectrochrome, he claimed, would cure all diseases by projection of colored light. Not ordinary light, of course, but rays from a 1,000-watt bulb passed through a glass tank of water and focused by a crude lens through colored glass slides. Spectrochrome promised something special—"No diagnosis, no drugs, no manipulation, no surgery"—simply "attuned color waves." The light boxes bore labels stating they were "for the measurement and restoration of the human radioactive and radio-emanative equilibrium."

Directions for the treatment were spelled out in Ghadiali's textbook titled, "Spectrochrometry." Combinations of light colors were specific for body areas and diseases being treated. Time of treatment was determined by the phases of the moon and the dictates of astrology. Latitude and longitude of the place of treatment were determined according to "solar, lunar and terrestrial gravitation." The patient had to be nude, with his body facing north.

A three-volume "Ghadiali Encyclopedia" defined the technical language of Spectrochrometry and contained case histories of people who were supposedly helped by it. "For legal protection," the Encyclopedia suggested that words like "imbalance" be used for "disease" and "normalate" for "cure."

Appropriate for an astrological society, followers of the cult were organized in local congregations called "planets." Each planet was headed by a "Normalator" who gave treatments and instructed the faithful. Spectrochrome was more than colored light séances—it was a way of life to its followers! They must eat no meat and use no alcohol, tea, coffee or tobacco. Honey and eggs were likewise taboo. Membership cost $90.00. Most amazing was the growth of the cult. At the time of the trial, Ghadiali had some 9,000 followers who paid dues and many others who took "treatments."

Pathos and tragedy marked the trial in Federal court at Camden, New Jersey, where victims of the fraud and survivors of other victims told their stories. The saddest testimony concerned people who had abandoned rational medical treatment and then succumbed to their diseases while depending on Spectrochrome.

Extremely pathetic were the "case histories" Ghadiali had published in his Encyclopedia. The Government presented five of these cases in court and proved that the allegedly successful results were false. Three of the victims died from the conditions Ghadiali claimed to have cured—two from tuberculosis, and a third from complications following severe burns. In the third case, the Encyclopedia contained photographs purporting to show the stages in the healing of burns that covered a little girl's body. The mother testified that scars and open sores had continued until the girl died. The fourth case was that of a girl whose sight Ghadiali claimed to have "restored," but who in fact was still totally blind. The fifth victim, a spastic girl completely paralyzed from the waist down, was carried to the witness chair. She had been photographed standing alone and reported to walk unaided. She testified that she had been supported by others except at the moment the picture was snapped.

Most dramatic was the testimony of the son of a man who died from diabetes. Pointing at the defendant, he charged: *"You told my father to stop insulin. You told him to eat plenty of brown sugar and starches. You said he would recover with Spectrochrome!"*

The evidence showed that Ghadiali himself did not believe in Spectrochrome. Certainly he was aware of the importance of suitable "qualifications" and had obtained a false M.D. degree from a diploma mill at a cost of $133.33. Other "degrees" were secured in a similar manner. One institution which he did attend was the Atlanta Penitentiary where he matriculated in 1925 after being convicted for violating the Mann Act.* (He said he was "framed" by the Ku Klux Klan.) Testifying in the 1930's against the passage of the Federal Food, Drug and Cosmetic Act, he claimed to have a million-dollar business.

The 42-day trial was the longest in the history of the FDA up to that time. Ghadiali had 112 witnesses who testified they had used Spectrochrome successfully, making a total of 216 persons whose cases figured in the trial. Government witnesses included experts on cancer, diabetes, tuberculosis, heart disease, blood pressure and nervous and mental disorders. The Government had to prove beyond a reasonable doubt that

---

* A U.S. law (1910) prohibiting transportation of women across state lines for immoral purposes.

Spectrochrome was a fraud and Ghadiali its perpetrator.

On January 7, 1947, the jury brought in a verdict of guilty on all 12 counts in the case. The sentence, by Federal Judge Philip Forman, was carefully designed to avoid making a martyr of Ghadiali and to put a stop to his gigantic swindle. This was accomplished through a $20,000 total fine, probation for five years, and a three-year prison term to be served if the defendant resumed his illegal activities.

On the very day his probation ended, Dinshah Ghadiali announced his intention to found a new "Institute." Changing the name slightly, he built more machines and resumed leadership of the local branches, renamed "studios." New literature was issued bearing substantially the same unwarranted claims as before. The FDA requested an injunction which became permanent in July 1958, finally ending the operations of this "colorful" cult.

An Endless Variety

The Spectrochrome was but one of literally hundreds of contraptions and gadgets which the FDA has dealt with since it first obtained legal powers over "therapeutic devices" in 1938. The extraordinary variety of these health fakes is in itself significant. They range from seemingly complex electronic instruments to disarmingly simple articles of everyday use.

One of the most amusing health fakes that I can recall was the Chiropra Therapeutic Comb, invented by Herr Dr. Theo. Schwarz, of Mannheim, Germany. Imports were spotted by U.S. Customs and turned over to FDA. It was the theory of Herr Schwarz that the act of scratching is beneficial, a well-known fact which he extended to extraordinary lengths. The Chiropra Comb, a soft rubber article with curved teeth, came with a

36-page illustrated manual of instructions on how to scratch—for the treatment of virtually all diseases. Charts showed the proper scratching patterns for men, women and children. For high blood pressure, for example, the instructions called for scratching the back of the trunk and the back of the lower legs. For arthritis deformans, criss-cross scratching of the lower back, and back of the left leg, was prescribed.

The Chiropra system was promoted in Germany by the "Chiropra Institute" of Heidelberg. FDA detained the imports on the basis of false claims that scratching would benefit such conditions as cancer, multiple sclerosis, asthma, heart and circulatory diseases, insomnia, constipation, lumbago, arthritis, stomachache, fallen arches and cold feet.

The variety of gadgets to cure anything and everything never ceases to amaze! But even more amazing is the uncritical capacity of so many people to believe that any one thing can do so much. About the same time that I heard of the Chiropra Comb (the mid-1950's), the FDA seized a little device called "Babylon's Zone Therapy Roller." This was simply a single large ball bearing mounted on a block of wood—resembling a furniture caster. The general idea was that massaging the feet on the ball could could be beneficial for many different conditions. After all, are not the feet connected to the rest of the body, and do they not affect the way you feel? So why not treat the whole body through the soles of the feet?

Speaking of combs reminds one of brushes and of Dr. Scott's Electric Hair Brush for the Bald. This turn-of-the-century marvel was warranted to cure nervous headache, bilious headache and neuralgia in five minutes! Over half a century later it took a hard-fought court case to stop a dentist's claims that regular use of his toothbrush kit was the best way to prevent heart disease, cancer, and birth defects in one's offspring!

Profits Vs. Consumer Protection

The Federal Food, Drug and Cosmetic Act of 1938 made it illegal to sell devices which are dangerous or are marketed with false claims. Fortunately, the word "device" is defined broadly so that the law covers any contrivance intended for therapeutic use. Unfortunately, the need to establish that devices are safe and effective *before they are marketed* was not appreciated in 1938. Thus, some manufacturers can and do put devices on the market with little or no effort to determine their safety or usefulness.

To remove a device from the market, the government must first know about it and then prove it to be dangerous or misrepresented. The more profitable the device, the more its promoters are likely to stretch out a court fight. Unless a device is clearly dangerous, it can usually continue to be sold until all court processes are ended.

A seemingly harmless device can turn out to be inherently dangerous. Consider the "Relax-A-Cisor," an electrical contraption for the overweight—designed to provoke muscle spasms through mild electrical shocks. This was promoted as "passive exercise," a pleasant and effortless way to reduce. It took years of investigation and a five-month court battle to put this profitable gismo out of business. Forty witnesses testified about the injuries they had received from its use. Medical experts explained the hazards of treatment with such a machine. Federal Judge William P. Gray summed up the evidence by saying the Relax-A-Cisor would be hazardous in a wide range of conditions including gastrointestinal, orthopedic, muscular, neurological, vascular, skin, kidney and female disorders. He found it could cause miscarriages and could aggravate such pre-existing conditions as epilepsy, hernia, ulcers and varicose veins.

More than 400,000 Americans fell for this major health hoax of the late 1960's. Obviously, to round up all these machines from all their users would have been practically impossible. Accordingly, the FDA issued a public warning and arranged for public notices to be displayed in U.S. Post Offices throughout the country.

Much gadget quackery is designed for use by health practitioners, especially chiropractors. During the 1950's and early 1960's, more than 5,000 "Micro-Dynameters" were sold. Chiropractors purchased most of them at prices up to $875.00. This machine was represented as capable of diagnosing and treating virtually all diseases (a sure sign of quackery). It consisted of a highly sensitive galvanometer fitted with various electrodes which were applied to different areas of the patient's body. Actually, the only condition it could detect was perspiration! Because of its uselessness, the Court of Appeals found the device unsafe even in the hands of a licensed practitioner. Announcing a nationwide campaign to round up all Micro-Dynameters in use, the FDA Commissioner called the machine "a peril to public health because it cannot correctly diagnose any disease." Thousands of people, he said, had been hoodwinked into believing they had diseases they did not have, or had failed to get proper treatment for diseases they did have.

Since 1972 the FDA has been carrying out a nationwide round-up of "Diapulse" devices. This machine was represented as an effective means of diathermy (deep heat) treatment. But FDA tests showed it produced an insignificant amount of heat—not enough for any therapeutic effect. Promoted mainly to M.D.'s,

230

Diapulse was backed by pseudomedical literature based on uncontrolled experiments. Many sales were made at seminars for doctors. During 1973 alone, more than 1,000 of the machines were seized or voluntarily turned over to the FDA.

The cost to patients of diagnosis or treatment with ineffective machines far exceeds the cost of the equipment. A conservative estimate would be $100 million annually.

Under the 1938 law, the FDA has concentrated on "quack" devices—generally those whose claims have greatly exceeded their performance. Devices designed for legitimate purposes, but which may be defective, have been left largely unregulated. Since the Government has the burden of proof, the manufacturer can put his device on the market and wait for the FDA to take action. Congress has been studying this problem for some years. Hopefully, a new comprehensive device law will be passed by the time this book is published.

From Witchcraft to Science Fiction

Since much gadget quackery is absurd, why do people fall for it?

Gadget quackery had its beginnings thousands of years ago when man first invented charms and fetishes to ward off evil spirits and cure disease. Belief in magic is still a major factor in the success of health fads and cults. At the same time, the miracles of science have made it easy to believe in science fiction.

When Benjamin Franklin published his discoveries on electricity he also helped open the door for two of the most famous frauds in medical history. The idea that this mysterious force might have medical applications was widely popular. Franklin himself had worked with a physician who attempted to use electric shock in treating a woman for convulsions. In 1784, while representing the United States in France, Franklin was appointed to a royal commission to investigate the hypnotist Antoine Mesmer, whose treatments had become the rage of Paris. Mesmer, clad in a lilac suit, carrying a metal wand and playing a harmonica, healed by what he called "animal magnetism." Patients sat around a huge vat or "battery," holding iron rods which were immersed in a solution. The treatments went on for hours, accompanied by shouts, hysterical laughter and convulsions. The Franklin commission, after conducting some experiments, reported no electricity in Mesmer's tub. Nor could they detect the current known as "animal magnetism." A royal decree banned further treatments, but Mesmer was allowed to take his winnings to England. On the commission besides Franklin were the noted chemist Lavoisier ("The Father of Modern Chemistry"), and a physician-inventor named Guillotin (the proposer of execution by beheading).

Ten years later, Elisha Perkins, a mule trader turned physician, secured a patent for "Perkins Tractors." Franklin was dead but popular interest in electricity was as great as ever. The tractors, two pointed rods about three inches long, one gold-colored, the other silver, were simply drawn downward across the afflicted part of the anatomy, in a sort of scratching motion. This, it was theorized, would draw off the "noxious fluid" (electricity) which was alleged to cause disease. "Tractoration," of course, was universal therapy—good for everything. For a time, the Perkins treatment enjoyed amazing popularity. Ministers, college professors and Congressmen gave enthusiastic endorsement. The Chief Justice of the Supreme Court bought a pair and President Washington himself is supposed to have been a customer. The medical profession was initially impressed; but in 1796 the Connecticut Medical Society condemned the treatment as "gleaned from the miserable remains of animal magnetism." In the following year the Society expelled Dr. Perkins from membership. In 1799, Dr. Perkins voluntarily served in a yellow fever epidemic in New York, caught the disease, and died. Tractoration withered away.

But electrical health gadgetry marched on—through the 19th century and into the 20th. Electric belts, peddled by pitchmen at county fairs, were credible because the magic of magnetism was being demonstrated in such marvels as the telegraph, the dynamo and the telephone. Then came the x-ray and radio, with accompanying waves of electronic quackery.

In the 1920's, Albert Abrams, M.D., invented the system of diagnosis and healing he called "Radionics." Soon more than 3,000 local practitioners, mainly chiropractors, were sending dried blood specimens from patients to be inserted in Abrams' "Radioscope." The diagnosis would come back on a postcard, with recommended dial settings for treatment with other Abrams machines.

Abrams left his lucrative business to the "College of Electronic Medicine" which he reportedly endowed with some $3 million to carry on his medical theories. The "college" was succeeded by the "Electronic Medical Foundation." When FDA agents investigated this business in the early 1950's, they looked first into the blood spot system of diagnosis. Inspectors arranged to send blood from an amputee and got back a report of arthritis in the right foot and ankle which the man had lost several years before. The blood of a dead man brought back a diagnosis of colitis, and that of an 11-week-old rooster resulted in a report of sinus infection and bad teeth!

Investigating the 13 different treatment machines, the FDA found just two basic types. The "Depolaray" and six other units simply produced magnetism from circuits like that of an electric doorbell. The "Oscillo-clast" and five similar machines had short-wave radio circuits resembling a taxicab transmitter. None could heal anything.

Officials of the Electronic Medical Foundation consented to a Federal court injunction in 1954, agreeing to stop all further promotion of the diagnostic system and devices. Shortly thereafter, they established the National Health Federation, an organization which would crusade against any government interference with quackery (see Chapter 13).

What made "Radionics" seem sensible to its victims? Certainly one factor was the experience of millions of Americans who had built homemade radios with crystal detectors and heard music in the earphones for the first time. Why couldn't blood crystals function like the crystal in the radio and reveal a person's diseases? Besides, hadn't their own trusted Dr. X taken the blood specimen and sent it away for analysis?

Treatment by Remote Control

Albert Abrams had many imitators, among them Ruth Drown, a Los Angeles chiropractor. One of her many nonsensical inventions was the Drown Radio-therapeutic Instrument. With this little black box and *two* blood spots, Mrs. Drown claimed to be able to "tune in" specific organs of the body and treat a patient by remote control anywhere in the world! When she was prosecuted by the FDA, one of the defense witnesses testified how she had been cured of pneumonia, from Hollywood, while attending a convention of the National Education Association in Atlantic City. When this witness was later identified by reporters as chairman of the Los Angeles Board of Education, there was an immediate reaction. How could someone so uninformed and gullible be in charge of the education of 400,000 children, be responsible for hiring science teachers, organizing health education programs, and the like? A resignation followed. Persons who are well-educated in some areas may be extremely naive in health matters.

Dr. Drown claimed that the only current used in her treatments was "the patient's own body energy." She alleged that tuning in on the "radio frequency" of the disease would automatically cause the disease cells to "fall away." Her followers were taught to conserve their "body magnetism." At the trial, one witness enthusiastically endorsed the Drown warning against shower baths. Since water was a conductor, his body magnetism and energy would go down the drain if he showered. In a tub bath, he was careful not to pull the stopper until he had climbed out, and to clean the tub with a long-handled brush!

The trial also had its tragic side. The Government's principal case history was that of a woman treated for breast cancer with the Drown device until her case became too advanced for successful surgery. Mrs. Drown was convicted and received the maximum fine of $1,000.

A Force Unknown to Science

"Unknown forces," as well as those familiar to science, have been exploited by the gadgeteers. William R. Ferguson combined both approaches in promoting his "Zerret Applicator."

More than 5,000 of these gadgets were sold to desperate, hopeful people throughout the Midwest in the late 1940's. Made of two blue and white plastic globes joined together (originally components of a baby rattle), the device was naturally nicknamed the "plastic dumbbell." Inside were two plastic tubes containing

"Zerret Water." Ferguson said this produced the "Z-ray, a force unknown to science." To have his diseases cured, a patient had only to sit holding the dumbbell, one ball in each hand, for at least 30 minutes at a time. The energy from the Z-rays would flow through the body and "expand all the atoms of your being." Directions warned not to cross the legs during treatment, since this could cause a "short circuit."

All this seems so ridiculous that one wonders why anyone would spend $50 for such a gadget. The reason seems to have been the timing of the promotion. The public was being informed about the wonders and possibilities of atomic energy. The *Chicago Tribune* had carried a series on the experiments at the University of Chicago involving plutonium and "heavy water," which led to the atom bomb. As in the time of Franklin and Perkins' tractors, people were hearing of possible health applications of a new kind of energy. The medical uses of x-rays were long established. Why shouldn't there be a Z-ray which could cure by its effects on the atoms of the body? Maybe it sounded silly, but why not give it a try? *It might work!* What did they have to lose? Only $50.

The medical con man Ferguson was sentenced to two years in Federal prison and a woman associate, Mary Stanakis, received a one-year sentence. Chemists proved at the trial that Zerret water was chemically identical to Chicago tap water.

During the same month, the Chicago Federal Court sentenced George Erickson and Robert Nelson to a year in prison for promoting the "Vrilium Tube" for radiation therapy. They recommended it for such conditions as cancer, diabetes, leukemia, thyroid disturbances, ulcers, arthritis and other serious conditions. This gadget was a brass tube two inches long, about as thick as a pencil, with a safety pin for attaching it to clothing.

Inside was a tiny glass tube filled with barium chloride, a chemical worth about $1/2000$ of a cent. It sold for $306.00, tax included.

Having to prove "beyond a reasonable doubt" that the Vrilium Tube was a fraud, the Government called some 35 witnesses, including distinguished atomic scientists, who established that the device was totally lacking in radioactivity and was worthless for any medical use. The most effective witness, however, was a man who described the death of his diabetic son who abandoned insulin and pinned his faith on the "Magic Spike."

Sentencing the defendants, Federal Judge Walter LaBuy said:

> "The sale of the device constitutes a gross fraud on the public . . . You have imposed on the poor sick who in their anxiety for relief would try anything at any price. You have fooled the trusting, the credulous and the gullible. The quackery you have employed is the more despicable because those who were deceived into believing in your fake remedy failed to pursue the treatment proven by medical science to be effective in preventing and curing diseases. This credulous belief in the efficacy of a useless product is the greatest danger inherent in quackery. It discourages and prevents those who use it from seeking proper medical treatment, and the results of such neglect are often fatal."

The Orgone Energy of Wilhelm Reich

Wilhelm Reich, M.D., one-time pupil of psychiatrist Sigmund Freud, claimed to have discovered "orgone energy," the most powerful force in the universe, and wrote extensively of its manifestations. Physical scientists, however, were unable to find the slightest evidence in Reich's data or elsewhere that such a thing as orgone exists.

Soon after coming to the United States in 1934, Reich designed and built "orgone accumulators." Most of them were boxes of wood, metal and insulation board about the size of a telephone booth. Disease, he claimed, could be cured simply by sitting inside the box and absorbing the orgone. Hundreds of the boxes were sold or leased to practitioners and laymen for treatment of all kinds of diseases including cancer. Rentals were around $250 per month. When the FDA sued in 1954 for an injunction to stop the hoax, Reich told the court that neither it, nor the FDA, would be capable of understanding his orgone science and therefore he would not offer a defense. The injunction was then issued on the basis of the Government's evidence. When Reich continued to promote the box for treating the sick, he was prosecuted for contempt of court. Found guilty, he was sent to prison where he died in 1956.

From the outset of his difficulties with the Government, Dr. Reich attempted to pose as a martyr and to make his case a *cause célèbre*. His family and followers have continued this effort. Destruction (by court order) of seized labeling material on the accumulator devices has produced accusations of "book burning." Actually, Reich's books have continued to be available. There has been no destruction of any of his publications other than those which accompanied the seized devices.

Scientology and Its E-Meter

Twenty years after the Spectrochrome trial, the FDA was again involved with a healing cult—"Scientology"—and a device used in its rituals, the "Hubbard Electropsychometer." The founder and the inventor of the "E-Meter" was a science fiction writer named Lafayette Ronald Hubbard. Hubbard has reportedly said: "If a man really wanted to make a million dollars, the best way would be to start his own religion."

Hubbard's original intention appears to have been merely to write an article for *Astounding Science Fiction,* a pulp magazine. Published in May 1950, the article was a hit—so much so that Hubbard dashed off a book-length version—*Dianetics: The Modern Science of Mental Healing.* Overnight, Dianetics became a popular fad. A Dianetic Research Foundation was established at Elizabeth, New Jersey. Practitioners trained by the Foundation set up offices in Hollywood, on Park Avenue and on Chicago's "Gold Coast." The practitioners were called "auditors" and patients were interviewed while they reclined on couches. After a few years, Dianetics declined in popularity, but the invention of the E-Meter and the incorporation of Scientology as a church, revived it.

FDA's involvement with Scientology began in 1958 when it learned that the Distribution Center of the organization was selling a drug called "Dianazine." This product was promoted for "radiation sickness," a condition widely feared at that time as a potential consequence of "fall-out" from atomic weapons testing. Dianazine, a vitamin mixture in tablet form, was seized and condemned by the court as misbranded.

A follow-up inspection led to an investigation of the E-Meter. Action against the device began when more than 100 E-Meters were seized by U.S. marshals at the headquarters of the "Founding Church of Scientology" in Washington, D.C. The court papers charged that the devices were misbranded by false claims that they treat effectively some 70 percent of all physical and mental illness. It was also charged that the devices did not

239

bear adequate directions for treating the conditions for which they were recommended in Scientology literature.

A jury trial resulted in a verdict that the E-Meter was misbranded by the Scientology literature—hence both the device and its "labeling" were subject to condemnation. The court rejected as irrelevant in this case the defense that the literature was exempt from legal action because it was issued by a "religious" organization. The Court of Appeals, however, reversed the verdict on the basis that the government had done nothing to rebut Scientology's claim that it was a religion. A new trial was ordered, at the close of which Judge Gerhardt A. Gesell issued a 14-page opinion. Regarding the practice of auditing, the judge said:

> "Hubbard and his fellow Scientologists developed the notion of using an E-Meter to aid auditing. Substantial fees were charged for the meter and for auditing sessions using the meter. They repeatedly and explicitly represented that such auditing effectuated cures of many physical and mental illnesses. An individual processed with the aid of the E-Meter was said to reach the intended goal of 'clear' and was led to believe that there was reliable scientific proof that once cleared many, indeed most, illnesses would successfully be cured. Auditing was guaranteed to be successful. All this was and is false—in short, a fraud."

Upholding FDA's charges that the E-Meter was misbranded, Judge Gesell ordered that use of the E-Meter be confined to "bona fide religious counseling" and that the device be prominently labeled with the warning notice:

"The E-Meter is not medically or scientifically use-

ful for the diagnosis, treatment or prevention of any disease. It is not medically or scientifically capable of improving the health or bodily functions of anyone."

After eight years of litigation, with two complete trials and three rulings of the Court of Appeals, the E-Meters and literature were returned to the Scientology headquarters. Was anything accomplished? Definitely, yes. The courts had seen the necessity to uphold the food and drug law even in a situation that involved the First Amendment. The court upheld the right of believers to believe—even in science fiction—provided that they do not violate the laws that protect the public health.

Don't Be Fooled!

How can you avoid being cheated by the gadgeteers and their gadgets? For they are still around in great variety in spite of legal efforts to combat them.

First and foremost, don't believe anyone who tells you that *one* kind of diagnosis or *one* kind of treatment is effective for a *wide range of diseases*. The ancient Greeks had a word for this kind of oversimplification— "panacea"—good for curing everything. All panaceas are quackery. Many of the devices discussed in this chapter belong in this category.

Beware of all gadgetry promoted to aid in reducing. All "passive" or "effortless" exercise machines are fakes. The same is true of massagers which are represented as capable of "spot reducing." There are no devices which can "reproportion" one's figure without dieting and proper exercise. That includes all so-called "body wraps" and other sweat-inducing garments, girdles, belts, etc.

Vibrator devices are on the market in great variety. Essentially for massage, they are often useful for temporary relief of muscular stiffness, aches and pains.

241

Excessive claims are often made for them, however. Vibrators are not effective for curing arthritis, rheumatism, nervous disorders, heart conditions and other serious diseases. Nor are they effective for reducing.

Youth, beauty and sex are constantly exploited by the gadgeteers, as well as by other quacks. Devices to enlarge and develop the female breast are hardy perennials in the garden of quackery. Typically, they are plastic cups which connect to a vacuum pump or water faucet to produce a massage effect. Dozens have been taken off the market by government action. They are not merely ineffective. If cancer cells are present, breast massagers can help them spread. Bust developers are usually sold by mail, and FDA collaborates with the U.S. Postal Service in prosecuting their promoters.

Drugs and devices for "lost manhood" are fakes. So are devices to enlarge the penis or support erection. Ads in cheap pulp magazines are the traditional medium for promoting this type of quackery. There are no devices in this category which fulfill their claims.

"Air purifiers" are sometimes promoted with excessive claims. Even ordinary household vacuum cleaners have been advertised as helpful in preventing allergies, hay fever and respiratory diseases. Although equipment does exist which can effectively remove dust and pollen, the small units sold by many firms are not able to do so. Because germ particles are so tiny, no air purifier can help prevent viral or bacterial diseases such as colds, influenza or pneumonia. "Negative ion generators" have no value in preventing or treating disease.

Summing Up

There are no machines which can diagnose or treat many different kinds of illnesses by applying electrical

242

contacts to the body, turning knobs and reading dials. Such devices are fakes!

Beware of gadgetry used by faith healers or promoted by crusading groups of laymen.

Don't fall for "science fiction." The miracles of legitimate medicine are much more wonderful and deserving of confidence.

If you suspect a gadget is misrepresented, don't hesitate to contact your nearest Food and Drug Administration office.

Last, do not assume that because an article is on the market, is advertised, is prescribed, or is sent through the mail, that it must be legitimate. Pre-marketing approval is not required for devices as it is for new drugs. And even if tougher device laws are enacted, as seems likely, they could not, of course, be entirely effective.

Editors' Note:

As Mr. Janssen predicted, a device bill became law in May, 1976, which will greatly increase the FDA's ability to combat device quackery.

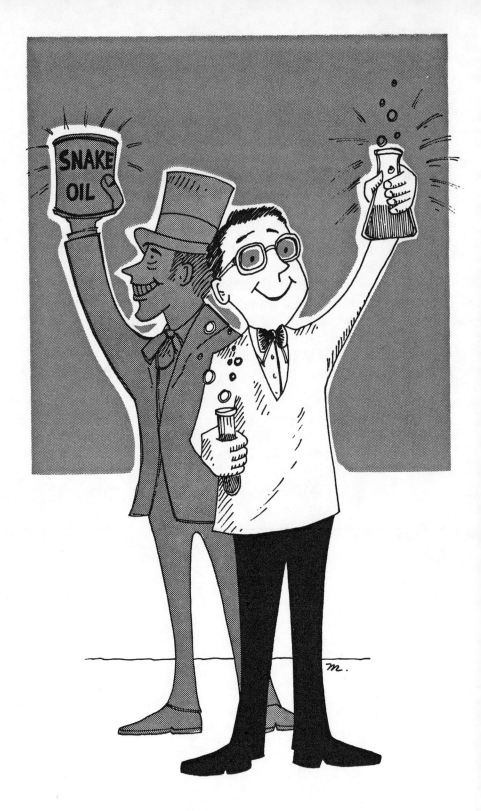

17

DUBIOUS DENTISTRY

The spread of questionable dental methods is a problem which is affecting many dentists and their patients today. Although this problem is serious, the dental profession has not yet developed an effective way to control it.

BY

WILLIAM T. JARVIS, Ph.D.
*Associate Professor of Preventive
and Community Dentistry
Loma Linda University School of Dentistry*

"I've had it!" Bob announced to his fellow dentists and luncheon companions, George and Jack. "I've been a dentist for nearly ten years and what have I really accomplished? Sure, I have a beautiful house, a boat, a motor home and a couple of cars. But what have I done for my patients? I fix them up and pretty soon they're back with more problems."

"I know what you mean," replied Jack. "Day in and day out a guy does dental work only to see the same problems repeating themselves. Wouldn't it be great if we could not only treat a patient's present dental problems, but also teach him how to avoid future ones."

"Yeah! That's what I think," returned Bob. "And not only that," he added, "we need to be more concerned about out patients' total health—not just their dental problems."

Feeling his enthusiasm start to rise, Jack continued, "I've been talking to some guys who have been doing just that! They've expanded their dental practice into a total health clinic which deals with the patient as a whole person. They do all kinds of tests, get into nutrition counseling, exercise, the whole bit! They're more than just dentists—they're really going after changing the total life style of their patients."

"Wait a minute, you guys," interrupted George who had been quietly taking in all that his colleagues were saying. "I'll agree that dentistry can become routine and a bit frustrating at times, but dentistry is still dentistry. I've heard about the dental practice you're talking about, Jack. I know for a fact that those guys are doing a lot of things which are beyond the scope of dentistry. Not only that, a number of things they're doing are pretty questionable scientifically. I'd think twice before getting involved in that sort of thing."

The three dentists were discussing the spread of questionable dental methods—a problem which is affecting many dentists and their patients today. Although this problem is serious, the dental profession has not yet developed an effective way to control it.

The Spread of Misinformation

Not all techniques used by dentists are learned at dental schools. New ideas and techniques are constantly being developed. Dentists who have graduated learn of these in various ways. One of the most common is by going to seminars conducted by other practitioners. Unfortunately, the dental profession has not yet developed a system to evaluate the validity of new methods promoted in this way. Too often, a questionable practice must become a major issue before a scientific body like the American Dental Association Council on Dental Research is prompted to issue a guiding statement. By that time, its promoters may have a following of dentists who will continue their practices even in the face of ADA recommendations to the contrary.

Information can also spread by word-of-mouth. Frank had been in dental practice for nine years when he bumped into an old schoolmate. "Vitamin E seems to help the gums," his friend said. "Just have your patients chew up a capsule, swish the remains around in their mouths, and floss them between their teeth." When Frank tried it, he thought he could see an improvement and his patients thought so, too. He would ask them such questions as, "Have you noticed that your gums aren't as red as they used to be?" or, "Do your gums bleed less now?" or, "Have you noticed less soreness?"

But some tricky things can happen when a clinician looks for something as subtle and subjective as changes in color and pain. Both patient and doctor tend to see what they hope to find. More important, when improvement does occur, people tend to credit the treatment even though a natural healing process may be responsible. There was a time in medical history when conclusions based upon simple observation were accepted because doctors didn't know better. Clinical observations are still a source of research leads. But with today's more sophisticated science, we know that such data are not trustworthy and must be backed by scientifically designed studies.

A true scientist will base his beliefs on an objective review of the data. His commitment should not be to his current beliefs, but to the pursuit of truth. If he receives better evidence, he should be able to change his position. But some people arrive at their beliefs through *delusion*. This means having preconceived theories which are fixed—so that new knowledge is either altered to fit one's theories or rejected as false. While the true scientist will change his theories of reality to bring them in line with the facts, the deluded investigator will change the facts to fit his theories!

Unfortunately, the deluded or misguided dentist doesn't wear a sign around his neck proclaiming himself to be unorthodox. Nor do his eyeballs give him away by rolling around in opposite directions. Steve Warmheart has been a dentist for fifteen years. He likes what he is but feels that most people do not appreciate just how important dentistry is. He firmly believes that the mouth is the barometer of total body health and that problems in the mouth are not just local but involve the patient's entire system. Steve relates everything he learns about health to this basic principle. Always a persuasive speaker, he can argue convincingly. No one can change his mind because he is so sure that his fundamental belief is correct. Unhappily, just that—his resistance to change—makes him untrustworthy as a scientist.

Many people believe that the actions of quacks are so preposterous that any thinking person (which we all regard ourselves to be) could easily spot them. This is a fallacy. The dubious dentist is apt to be more personable and charming than is usual. Often he will do an exceptional job of selling himself to his patients. While friendliness, personal concern and charm are not good reasons to be suspicious of a dentist, neither do such traits assure the legitimacy of his theories.

Now let us look at some questionable practices.

Nutritional Pseudoscience

Balancing Body Chemistry. A number of dentists have been touring the country promoting the notion of "balancing body chemistry" by nutritional methods. These men toss biochemical concepts about quite freely in their seminars. Unfortunately, most dentists exposed to their theories do not have the scientific expertise to recognize the falsity of their claims. As a result, nutrition nonsense has been making inroads into the thinking of many dentists. The problem is compounded by the fact that many of these seminars are sponsored by dental organizations—sometimes even for "continuing education" credit. (That means official recognition such as credit toward relicensure requirements.)

The general hope of balancing body chemistry is that dietary practices can prevent a wide variety of "degenerative" diseases. Special diets and expensive food supplements are recommended to achieve "balance," and various laboratory tests are used to determine the biochemical state of the patient. Supporters of these methods greatly exaggerate what nutrition can do. Their patients are absorbing false hope and wasting money on lab tests and food supplements.

Organized dentistry has begun to speak out against this dubious practice. In December 1975, the ADA Council on Dental Research criticized the diet recommended by one of its leading promoters—Hal Huggins, D.D.S., of Colorado Springs, Colorado. The Huggins diet is of the high-protein, low-carbohydrate variety. Having reviewed the evidence with the aid of qualified consultants in the field of biochemistry and human metabolism, the Council concluded: "There is little or no evidence to support the broad claims of the Hal Huggins diet. . ."

Hair Analysis. Closely connected to balancing body chemistry is the technique known as hair analysis. Here a sample of hair is sent to a laboratory for spectrographic analysis. The laboratory report states which components are "deficient" and recommends specific supplements—often the lab's own brand. The practitioner then sells the product to the patient.

The AMA Committee on Cutaneous Health and Cosmetics recently issued a statement concerning the abuse of hair analysis. It pointed out that the state of the body's health may be completely unrelated to the chemical condition of the hair. Hair composition is affected by a person's age, sex and natural hair color. It is also affected by exposure to tonics, hair sprays, shampoos, environmental contaminants in the air, chlorine in swimming pools and so forth.

Hair analysis may have some use in detecting the presence of certain minerals, but it is of *limited* value in determining a person's nutritional state. The proper way to measure body stores of trace elements, as well as other nutrients, is by analysis of body tissues and fluids. You should be skeptical of dentists who use hair analysis as the basis for prescribing food supplements.

Computer Analysis. An insightful student of quackery once wrote: "Every new science, every fresh invention, has been capitalized to serve the needs of universal charlatanism. Quackery always takes its cues from the world of knowledge." Abuse of the computer is an excellent case in point. Many dentists are using computers to analyze the diets of their patients. As with the hair analysis scheme, the computer analysis usually leads to a recommendation of specific dietary supplements by brand name. While computer analysis of diet is an interesting concept, investigation has shown that most of its present applications are not reliable. You should be skeptical of dentists who offer this service as a means of prescribing food supplements.

The Anti-Sugar Crusade. Dentists will generally tell you that sugar is bad for your teeth. But research shows that the physical nature of foods and frequency of intake are even more important in producing tooth decay than is the amount of sugar that is eaten. Length of contact with the tooth's surface is the key factor. For this reason, honey, dried fruits, pastries and cereals—which can stick in the pits and fissures of teeth—are the foods most likely to produce cavities. Soda pop, a major sugar-containing product, doesn't have as great a decay-producing effect because it generally doesn't stay in contact with the tooth surface very long.

The dental profession has long sought to teach people not to eat sweets as snacks—especially sticky, gooey sweets. But some dentists seem to have an obsession about sugar and attack it with the fervor of evangelists. Many of these anti-sugar warriors have been influenced by the writings of Weston Price, an early 20th century dentist who imagined that sugar causes not only tooth decay, but physical, mental, moral and social decay as well.

Making a whirlwind tour of the places where primitive people could be viewed, Price examined them superficially and jumped to conclusions. Extolling their health, he overlooked their short life expectancy, high infant mortality, endemic diseases and malnutrition. Praising their diets for not producing cavities, he ignored the fact that malnourished people don't usually get many cavities.

251

Price pointed out that primitive people who had few cavities when they ate native food developed dental troubles when exposed to civilization. But he did not realize why. Most primitive people are used to "feast or famine" eating. When large amounts of sweets are suddenly made available, they overindulge themselves! Not knowing the value of balancing their diets, they also ingest too much salt and fatty foods.

Price also noted that exposure to civilization had led to an increased incidence of other diseases. But this increase was not caused simply by exposure to the food supply of the civilized world, as Price imagined. Diet was a factor—but it was not merely a matter of eating "civilized" food, but of *abusing* it. Price apparently overlooked other factors which were important in increasing the disease rate. One was exposure to unfamiliar germs, to which the natives were not resistant. Another was the drastic change in their way of life as they gave up strenuous physical activities such as hunting. Alcohol abuse was also a factor.

Today's anti-sugar warriors are highly philosophical in their approach. Many of them believe that dental problems are not caused by local factors in the mouth but are due to problems of the body as a whole. Though lacking evidence to support this idea, they talk as though they have discovered the Holy Grail! Some have even gone to the point of injecting insulin into the gums of their patients to "retard the activity of sugar around the teeth."

The anti-sugar dentists have found strong moral support in the world of the unorthodox and often become heroes to its believers. They are often the same dentists who make public statements against the proven benefits of fluoridation—suggesting instead that elimination of sugar from the diet is all that is needed to prevent cavities. Removing sugar from the diet is not a realistic suggestion—and even if this could be done, tooth decay would not be eliminated.

Dietary Treatment of Cancer. Like all of the health care professions, dentistry has individuals who abuse their dental degrees by promoting unorthodox methods for patients who are hopelessly ill. One such dentist is William D. Kelley who, for many years, operated a clinic and computer laboratory in Grapevine, Texas. Kelley believes that cancer is caused by "inadequate production or utilization of enzymes." In his book, *One Answer to Cancer*, he claims that cancer can be diagnosed by "simple urinalysis," that it "often can be controlled by diet alone," and that it can "almost always be controlled by proper dosage of enzymes."

Not long ago I interviewed a middle-aged woman who had consulted him. During surgery, doctors had discovered a large cancer of the pancreas which had spread to her liver. Feeling desperate, the woman turned to Dr. Kelley who ran a computer analysis of her case. His marvelous machine clicked out the information that her tumor was 50 months old, was growing, and was caused by a mineral deficiency. It would take 11 months to cure and 19 months to regain nutritional balance. The patient returned home with a booklet full of menus and several hundred dollars poorer—but loaded with hope.

After many years of difficulty with various federal and state law enforcement agencies, Kelley has reportedly left the State of Texas. His faulty notions continue to be promoted by his book and by organizations which promote unproven cancer cures.

Public Protection

Your primary protection from dubious dentistry should come from dental organizations at the local, state and national level. Unfortunately, not all of these groups have an effective means of screening out questionable practices *before* they have been foisted on the public. The American Dental Association Councils on Research and Therapeutics are working on this problem, and hopefully will find a solution in the near future.

Another source of accurate information should be the nation's dental schools. It is sad to report, however, that even a few schools have been caught up in the epidemic of delusion which is so rampant in dentistry. At the University of Alabama, for example, the Chairman of the Department of Oral Medicine is Dr. Emanuel Cheraskin, one of the most popular spokesmen of the health food movement (see Chapter 12).

Cheraskin's main message seems to be that nutrition is of tremendous value in preventing and treating diseases—especially those which are usually thought of as hopeless. He regards most physicians and dentists as ignorant about nutrition. Only he and other "nutritionally oriented" practitioners know what's really happening in the disease process. With folksy sarcasm, Cheraskin criticizes orthodoxy and praises megavitamin therapy. He feels that the food we eat is sadly devitalized as it goes from "garden to gullet," and that ideal nutrition is impossible without vitamin supplementation. He bases broad assumptions upon poorly conceived research and uses testimonials as evidence of the effectiveness of his nutrition programs.

In his latest book, *Psychodietetics,* Cheraskin admits that he has failed to convince most health professionals (who are qualified to evaluate his claims) and thus takes his case to the public where he expects a "more enthusiastic response." But his books are widely read by dentists, many of whom regard him as a hero.

We hope this chapter will help you as a consumer to recognize current situations in which your health or your pocketbook may be in jeopardy. We also hope that dentists who read this will become more wary of certain dental promoters. Recognizing quackery in all its forms is a formidable task for anyone. Its methods usually seem so honorable, its promoters so convincing. Its methods or materials may even have legitimate applications in some other ways. Sometimes the only dividing line between quackery and hopeful new ideas lies not in what is done, but in how much is promised by the doer.

Modern dentistry is striving for an ideal which places its highest priority on preventing dental diseases by identifying causes and teaching patients how to avoid them. The concept of treating the dental patient "as a whole person" is also rapidly gaining acceptance. Certainly, most dentists who talk about prevention are not promoting quackery. On the other hand, it is clear that many dentists are going overboard in reaching for these ideals.

The motives of such dentists are not necessarily in question. But good intentions are not enough. If dental science is to advance, it must patiently obey the strict rules by which all science advances. And if the profession of dentistry is to remain reputable, it must find a way to control the spread of dubious methods.

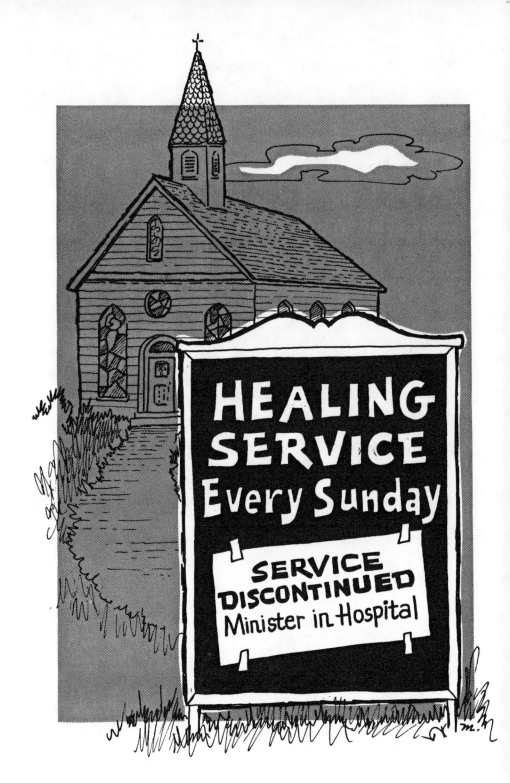

18

THE MIRACLE MERCHANTS

"The Power of Positive Greed"

BY
REV. LESTER KINSOLVING

Does Faith Healing Work?

Mary Vonderscher of Burbank, California, thought it did. She felt cured of cancer of the spine, she said, even though doctors had thought her case was hopeless. Appearing on an Oral Roberts TV spectacular in mid-1955, Mrs. Vonderscher gave a glowing testimonial. In January, 1956, relatives of hers in Indiana saw a re-run of this program—just three days before they went to California for her funeral.

Wanda Beach, another believer, was a 37-year old diabetic from Detroit. In 1959, after telephoning her mother that Roberts had "completely cured" her, she threw away her insulin. And died.

Though the faith of these two ladies did not appear to heal them, it is not difficult to understand it. Sick people are prone to reach desperately for hope—especially when it is presented in a convincing way. And Oral Roberts could be quite convincing. When he rolled his mighty baritone into overdrive and howled, *"HEAL LORD!"* neither the Almighty nor the ailing appeared able to resist him. *"DO YOU FEEL HEALED?"* he would bellow—as if anyone submitting to such a scenario would dare to say no!

Roberts' enthusiasm for his work was unbounded. He moved into the big time with the skilled coaching of J. L. White, the same publicity expert who launched ultra-right wing anti-Communist Christian crusader Billy James Hargis.

The Jesuit magazine *America,* in a critique of Roberts entitled *Faith Healing over T.V.,* noted: "There is certainly a reasonable doubt that these programs are in the public interest. Of their very nature, they play on the hopes and fears of the credulous and ignorant. There is no positive proof that some of the 'cures' are not rigged. At any rate, standard medical treatment seems to be flouted. We can wonder how many, viewing such programs in their homes, are impelled to neglect ordinary medical treatment."

Nobody knows how many. It is not customary for faith healers to keep medical statistics.

In 1966, Roberts began a rather spectacular transition from Pentecostal Holiness to Methodist—leaving behind the faithful who had launched his healing ministry with many thousands of their dollars. He stopped broadcasting in May 1967. The following year he joined the Boston Avenue Methodist Church in Tulsa, Oklahoma. Although he had previously been quoted as saying: "I consider Hollywood and all its works unclean," in March, 1969, he reappeared on TV—in Hollywood.

His new programs are straight evangelism—a Sunday series plus quarterly prime time specials—all broadcast from the same unclean Hollywood. He is also owner and President of Oral Roberts University, whose 500 acre, $30 million campus is located in Tulsa. O.R.U.'s basketball team, one of the finest money can buy, is apparently a high priority item. In a *Sport* magazine article, basketball player Dana Lewis told what happened when he wanted to transfer to the University of Tulsa: "When they heard I was thinking of leaving, one of the vice-presidents of O.R.U. got in touch with my mother, who is very religious. He said he had just talked with the Lord and He'd said it was His will that I stay at O.R.U."

As far as I know, Roberts no longer specializes in healing. When I visited O.R.U.'s campus, it had an M.D. on its staff and all students were required to have health insurance.

Kathryn The Great

After Roberts shifted from the healing circuit to Hollywood, his place was immediately taken by Kathryn

("The Great") Kuhlman, a spectacular successor to the late Aimee Semple McPherson. Kathryn's Friday morning services jammed the spacious First Presbyterian Church in Pittsburgh. When I covered one of them, I saw busloads of people from seven states.

Kathryn skipped onto the stage, her golden sheath dress, red hair, pearly teeth and blue eyes all glistening in the spotlights. For five hours—without a break—this dynamic woman was on her feet preaching, praying, leading hymns, laying on hands and cheerleading, for God as well as every one of the hundreds who announced that they had been healed. As the healed came forward (often healing presumably took place en route from seat to platform), Kathryn would walk with them or direct them:

"Bend down, honey (and prove your arthritis has vanished)." Or, "Run down the aisle and show everybody you're healed!" Loudly thanking the Holy Spirit, Kathryn would clutch each miracle recipient—and then push him so he fell into the arms of a ready (and agile) assistant.

When the pace of miracles slackened, Miss Kuhlman would give The Spirit a nudge. Beaming those beautiful eyes heavenward, she would become psychic. "Someone in the balcony has just been cured of asthma!" Or, "There is someone who has just recovered his hearing!" (At this point, two elderly men jumped up, waved their earphones madly and shouted that they were no longer deaf.) At another point, Miss Kuhlman cried out: "I can feel it! Someone in the rear needs help, because he is wearing a truss!" (But nobody responded.)

Kathryn was advertised as "an ordained Baptist minister." But during an interview, she admitted that she had no theological education prior to receiving "honorary recognition" from something called "Evangelical Church Alliance, Inc.," of Joliet, Illinois.

Her formal education ended after two years of high school in Missouri when her father died. At age 16, and looking better than Susan Hayward, she persuaded a group of Baptist deacons in Twin Falls, Idaho, to let her fill a vacant pulpit. One of the deacons was sufficiently sophisticated to call the local press photographer. Her first scheduled sermon jammed the church to overflow.

While much of her oratorical style and humor was pure corn on the cob, Miss Kuhlman was much smarter than most faith healers. Instead of ignoring or attacking the medical profession, she used it—knowing that there are some Fundamentalist M.D.'s who will "certify" miracles without checking up on them afterward. One such doctor is Martin Biery, M.D., a retired surgeon from Garden Grove, California. During nine years of sitting regularly on Kathryn's platform, Dr. Biery saw dozens of "miracles" which he had not bothered to research.

Why not?

"I guess it's because of my faith in God and my trust in Him and my belief in Kathryn as a vessel of His that I don't worry about it. I feel, let the Lord take care of it."

A Troubled Year

The year 1975 produced a sea of troubles for Kathryn. First, William Nolen, M.D., a surgeon from Minnesota, exploded her certification gimmick in his book, *Healing: A Doctor in Search of A Miracle*. Dr. Nolen, who is not a Fundamentalist, was able to record the names of 25 people who were "miraculously healed" by Kathryn at a service in Minneapolis. When he followed up these cases later, he found among other things that one lady with Hodgkin's disease had been announced by Kathryn as cured of lung cancer—but the Hodgkin's disease remained unaffected. Another woman with cancer of the spine had thrown off her brace and followed Kathryn's joyful command to run across the stage. The following day her backbone collapsed and four months later she died. Overall, not one patient with organic disease had been helped.

Dr. Nolen's disastrous disclosures were followed by an internal explosion which was picked up by *People* magazine. Paul Bartholomew, Kathryn's former personal administrator, filed a $430,000 damage suit. Bartholomew, who said he had been paid $2,500 per week in commissions plus a $15,000 annual salary, charged Miss Kuhlman with breach of contract.

At the same time she fired Bartholomew, another Kuhlman mainstay, pianist Dino Kartsonakis, was replaced. Dino disclosed that the faith healer's announced income from the Kathryn Kuhlman Foundation ($25,000 a year) was augmented by a "walk-in vault" in the basement of her suburban mansion near Pittsburgh which contained more than $1 million worth of jewelry and another $1 million in art works. ("As God is my judge," Kathryn told this writer, "that isn't so. You're perfectly free to visit and inspect my home.")

Los Angeles magazine published an even more devastating exposé. For it was in Los Angeles that Kathryn taped her syndicated TV shows—and packed the Shrine auditorium.

"EACH MONTH, WHEN KATHRYN KUHLMAN HITS TOWN, THE LORD MAKES THE LAME TO WALK, THE DEAF TO HEAR—AND THE COFFERS TO SWELL," headlined a story by Jeanie Kasindorf.

"It isn't my ministry, she says, *He has given everything . . . I have actually given my life! (A long pause.) My body!"*

Writer Kasindorf concluded: "Now that, I say to myself, is a sermon that Burroughs Waltrip, Jr., would love to hear. Because Burroughs Waltrip last saw his father in 1936 when he was eight years old, when his father ran off with a lady evangelist named Kathryn Kuhlman."

Kathryn The Great managed to recover from this scandal, which disintegrated her fast-growing Denver Revival Tabernacle in 1936. In 1970, during an interview, I asked her: "Does the name Burroughs A. Waltrip mean anything to you?"

"How did you know?" she gasped. "He was the best-looking guy that ever was!" But "he was divorced and I had to choose between him and my work."

Ever since the worship of Venus, the sex-and-salvation formula has been achieving spectacular results—but hardly if the sex goddess is married to a handsome and virile man. During a telephone interview, Miss Kuhlman recalled that the last time she saw Burroughs Waltrip was in the Los Angeles railroad station in 1938. "He told me if I got on that train, I'd never see him again," she said.

Despite these shocks, Kathryn carried on her work. She seemed absolutely tireless and had an iron will and a positively hypnotic charm. She settled out of court with ex-administrator Bartholomew for an undisclosed amount. "It's much less than he asked for," she told me. "I found he was writing a book called *The Late Great Kate*. I am very much alive!" Then she added: "You reporters seem to know just about everything. But I love you just the same!"

In December, 1975, Kathryn entered a Tulsa, Oklahoma, hospital for open heart surgery. Though she survived the operation, she died on February 20, 1976.

The Power of Positive Greed

The financial successes of Oral Roberts and Kathryn Kuhlman have spurred a vaste horde of imitators. Two of the best known are Asa Alonzo Allen (A. A. Allen of Miracle Valley, Arizona) and Frederick J. Eikerenkoetter II ("Reverend Ike" of Harlem's United Church Center).

Allen, who bore a striking resemblance to the late zany bandleader Spike Jones, died on June 11, 1970, in the Jack Tar Hotel in San Francisco—of what his Miracle Valley associates solemnly announced as: "Apparently a heart attack." But U.P.I. subsequently reported that according to City Coroner Henry Turkel, faith-healer Allen died of "acute alcoholism and fatty infiltration of the liver."

A. A. Allen managed to survive several less serious crises. After switching from Methodist to Pentecostal as a boy, he was unfrocked by the Assemblies of God after being arrested for drunken driving in Knoxville, Tennessee. In another crisis, Allen settled out of court after being sued for $500,000 by the Freethinkers of America because he said their teachings "coincide perfectly with the methods taught by Communists."

On occasion, Allen's assistants would exclude newspaper reporters from his healing services, even as he furiously denounced the press. In Cleveland, *The Plain Dealer* exposed the fact that Allen had been charged with drunkenness in Laguna Beach, California, and in Las Vegas.

In 1962, Allen filed suit for divorce from his wife Lexie, asking the court to stop her from filing insanity proceedings against him—for the third time.

But while referring to himself as "The World's Most Persecuted Preacher," Allen made a statement which apparently became a creed to Reverend Ike: "As far as I am concerned, those who die in poverty, die in shame."

Rev. Ike, a virile clotheshorse of the Liberacean school of dress, elaborates upon this theme in his nationwide broadcasts and crusades—as well as in Harlem's Palace Auditorium. He regularly fills all 5000 seats of this auditorium, while proclaiming what *Time* magazine diagnosed as "The Power of Positive Greed."

Screams Rev. Ike to his ecstatic flocks: "I can love the Lord a lot better when I've got money in my pocket! Bless money! God is money in action! Now I'm about to pray the prayer of success and prosperity. And as I pray, I'm going to receive the evening's offering. I don't want everyone to give—only those who see themselves as having greater prosperity . . . Hold those bills high! I want everyone to see your faith!"

Complications

Physicians recognize that the power of faith may affect the condition of sick people. But such faith can work two ways. Although healers can "really give you a mental lift," there are other reactions which the faithful can have. Believers who are not helped may blame themselves. They may become sicker or severely depressed by such contemplations as: *"Faith always heals; I'm not healed; I'm being punished! What have I done wrong? What's wrong with me?"*

The medical profession does not believe that "faith healing" can cure people who have *organic* disease—that is, disease which changes the structure of parts of the body. After two vigorous years of tracking down "miracles," Dr. Nolen did not find a single one.

But many diseases are *functional,* wherein emotions play a large part in causing symptoms. Functional ailments can sometimes be relieved by the ministrations of a faith healer—or for that matter by the reassurance of a medical doctor. The big problem with faith healers of all types is that they do not know their limitations. Untrained in medical diagnoses, they rarely even try to distinguish between those cases they may be able to help and those which are beyond their ability.

In some cases, too much faith can be lethal:

—In Toronto, potential faith healer Mark Cowen explained to a coroner's jury that he had hoped to use his 20-year old wife as an exhibit of a "miracle cure" and had thrown away her insulin.

—In Barstow, California, in 1973, Mr. & Mrs. Lawrence Parker followed the advice of a visiting evangelist to stop giving insulin to their 11-year old son, Wesley. When the boy died as a result, the Parkers and 200 other people attracted national attention by refusing to allow burial for six days—because, they assured everyone, the evangelist had said resurrection was imminent. Subsequently found guilty of manslaughter, the Parkers were placed on probation with a requirement that they consult with a psychiatrist.

—In Van Nuys, California, in 1954, school teacher Cora Louise Sutherland died of tuberculosis after having exposed thousands of school children to the disease—because she had refused, as a Christian Scientist, to have an x-ray examination. Instead, according to *TIME* magazine, she resorted to a Christian Science practitioner who charged her $65 a month to "treat" her with prayer and readings from Mary Baker Eddy.

The "Science of Prayer"

Mary Baker Glover Patterson Eddy was a native of New Hampshire. She was an ardent admirer and disciple of Phineas Parkhurst Quimby, a faith healer and "metaphysician" from Maine. Her first husband, Gilbert Glover, died of fever. Left pregnant, penniless and very sick, she proceeded to marry her dentist, Daniel Patterson, whom she later divorced on charges of desertion. Finally she married Asa Gilbert Eddy, ten years her junior, a mild-mannered man who served her devotedly as she expanded the movement which she called "Christian Science."

In 1882, husband Asa Eddy died of valvular heart disease—but Mrs. Eddy called in the press to announce that he had been "murdered by arsenic mentally administered by malicious mental practitioners" whom she identified as three of her alienated pupils.

Among Mrs. Eddy's teachings was the idea that dead individuals continue to live "even though unseen by persons on our planes of existence." She also taught that prayer could heal, even at considerable distances. The January, 1976, *Christian Science Journal* lists about 4,300 practitioners who are licensed by The Mother Church (of Boston) to do healing.

According to a recent publication of the Christian Science Publishing Society, "Every student of Christian Science has the God-given ability to heal the sick."

Citation of the Cora Sutherland case in my nationally syndicated column evoked a number of protests. One came from Rollin E. Mayer of the Christian Science Committee on Publications for Indiana—whose function, according to the *Yearbook of American Churches,* is to correct "in a Christian manner, impositions on the public in regard to Christian Science."

Said Mayer: "Mr. Kinsolving . . . refers in a wholly misleading way to Christian Science. It seems unnecessary therefore to state that Christian Scientists are law-abiding and responsible members of the community . . . They report all communicable diseases . . . any Christian Scientist known to be suffering from a communicable disease would naturally report it."

My column had not mentioned that three of the nation's best-known Christian Scientists are H. R. Haldeman, John Erlichman and Emil Krogh. Nor had it mentioned the case of Christian Scientist Dorothy Sheridan who was found guilty by a Massachusetts jury of contributing to the death of her five year old daughter. In 1967, when the girl contracted pneumonia, Mrs. Sheridan reported it all right—but not to medical authorities. She reported it to a Christian Science practitioner, who prayed—while the child died.

On October 19, 1972, the Connecticut State Department of Health was told of a suspected polio outbreak at the Daycroft School, a Christian Science boarding and day school in Greenwich. The report came not from the school authorities but from a physician in Greenwich. Investigation by Dr. DeWayne Andrews of the Health Department revealed that the first child had become ill on September 29. When tests confirmed the diagnosis of polio, Dr. Andrews ordered a quarantine. He also ordered mass immunization of the 128 students and 35 faculty (a number of whom complained that this compromised their Christian Science faith).

Eleven youngsters suffered varying degrees of paralysis. Five of them were sent home—where they could expose others to this terrible disease. The other victims were sent to the school infirmary—where, it was explained to Dr. Andrews: "A compound fracture can be healed with 30 minutes of prayer."

Dr. Andrews contacted another Christian Science school, Principia, in St. Louis, to discuss the possibility of a similar epidemic. He recalls: "They wouldn't even discuss the subject." Neither would the national headquarters of the Committee on Publications, at Christian Science's Mother Church in Boston, when I telephoned to inquire.

The Christian Science headquarters also refused to disclose either its financial records or its membership figures. I suspect, though, that Church membership is on the decline—that today's young people are simply not buying its doctrines. In Malden, Massachusetts, stands the First Church of Christ Scientist, founded by Mary Baker Eddy herself. Built to seat 600, it had just 35 people present on Sunday morning, June 3, 1973.

Only three of these looked under 60 or 70—a virile young (paid) soloist and two obviously interested young girls peering at him from the front row.

Using volunteer reporters, I was able to survey all seven Christian Science Churches in Washington, D.C., at 11 A.M. on Sunday, January 26, 1976. Total seating capacity is more than 2,500. Attendance was about 500, with fewer than 25 appearing to be under age 60.

The number of practitioners listed in *The Christian Science Journal* has declined 13% in the past five years and fifty fewer churches are listed. When a church goes defunct and is sold, where does the money go? Allison Phinney, at the denomination's new $70 million headquarters building in Boston, said he didn't know. But Catherine Chance, of San Francisco's Northern California Committee on Publications, said she believes that all such proceeds revert to the Mother Church in Boston.

The Mother Church's self-perpetuating five-man Board of Directors conceals the finances from both the public and the contributing membership. It has been revealed, however, that *The Christian Science Monitor* lost $5 million in 1972—while in 1973, for the first time, the Board of Directors elected a foreign Treasurer, Marc E. Engeler.

Mr. Engeler is a Swiss banker.

PART TWO
The Struggle—To Protect Your Money and Your Life

19

THE TRUTH-SEEKERS

Throughout the world, hundreds of thousands of scientists work continuously to determine the boundaries of scientific thought. So if you find someone referred to as a "scientist ahead of his time," he is probably a quack.

BY

STEPHEN BARRETT, M.D.
Chairman, Board of Directors
Lehigh Valley Committee Against Health Fraud, Inc.

One way to avoid being robbed of cash and health is to get good information when you need it. Most of this book will tell you about people who can cheat you because they are confused or crooked. In this chapter, let's talk about where you can get honest, true and accurate answers to your health questions.

First, what is meant by "truth" in medical science and how is it determined?

Mankind has always been curious about disease and what causes it. The more we understand, of course, the better we can control illness. Down through the centuries, countless people have shared their observations and ideas. Thousands of theories have been offered to explain what men saw. During the past century, however, ideas have developed which seem to make more sense than others before them. And armed with these ideas, man has been able to prevent and cure diseases in an almost miraculous fashion.

As part of this process of scientific development, good methods have developed to test whether theories are logical. The sum of these methods is known as the "experimental" or "scientific" method. This method is used to answer questions like: "If two things happen, are they related?" For example, suppose you take vitamin E when you have a headache and the headache goes away. How can we tell whether the vitamin relieved you or whether the headache would have gone away by itself anyway? Throughout the world, hundreds of thousands of scientists work continuously to determine the boundaries of scientific thought.

As mountains of information are collected, how can we tell which evidence is valid? "Valid" means honestly collected and properly interpreted—using good techniques of statistical analysis. One hallmark of a good experiment is that others can repeat it and get the same results.

272

This brings us to the question of who can interpret experimental findings. Scientists are judging each other all the time. People with equal or superior training look for loopholes in experimental techniques and design other experiments to test conclusions. Skilled reviewers also gather in groups whose level of ability far exceeds that of the average scientist. Such experts are not likely to be misled by poorly designed experiments. Among the reviewers are editors and editorial boards of scientific journals. These people carefully screen out invalid findings and publish significant ones. As good ideas are put to use, more reports are generated. Gradually, a shared set of beliefs is developed which is felt to be scientifically accurate. When we speak of the "scientific community," we refer to this overall process of separating what is scientific fact from what is not.

Quacks, of course, operate outside of the scientific community. They do not use the scientific method to evaluate what they see. In fact, they seldom bother to experiment at all. Quacks try to cover up their inadequacies by pointing out that the scientific community has made mistakes in the past. This, of course, is true. But in recent years, the chances of major error by the scientific community have decreased greatly. So if you find someone referred to as a "scientist ahead of his time," he is probably a quack!

Six major types of agencies digest scientific information about health:

1. Health Professional Groups

The American Medical Association is still the most comprehensive source of good medical information. It does little clinical research, but does a great deal of evaluating. Through its various divisions, departments and committees, the AMA provides physicians with information on almost every aspect of the practice of medicine. It publishes eleven journals and many books and pamphlets. It has a service through which any physician can get an individual answer to his medical questions from top medical experts. It oversees a wide variety of educational programs for physicians. As a direct service to the public, for many years it published *Today's Health*—a fine monthly magazine which contained news of medical developments, articles on health care and disease, and answers to commonly asked questions.

Some of the political activities of the American Medical Association have been criticized as self-serving. Its scientific and educational activities are outstanding, however, and have been a big factor in the advance of health care in this country. The American Dental Association, American Osteopathic Association, American Psychiatric Association, American Dietetic Association and American Podiatric Association are among the groups which provide similar services for their respective professions.

2. Government Agencies

Many state and federal agencies evaluate scientific data and furnish information to consumers. The United States Public Health Service evaluates information which applies to public health. The National Institutes of Health undertake research. The Office of Consumer Affairs answers questions on a wide variety of topics. The Food and Drug Administration monitors food and drug safety. Its publication, *FDA Consumer*, lists government health fraud prosecutions and contains articles about health, safety and nutrition. (Subscription information can be obtained from the Superintendent of Documents, Government Printing Office, Washington, D.C. 20402.)

3. Medical Schools, Colleges, Universities and Other Training Centers

Most medical research is done at centers where doctors are trained. Such centers also help practicing physicians keep up-to-date.

4. Scientific Organizations and Publications

Many independent groups evaluate data and publish reports and journals. *The Medical Letter* furnishes physicians with excellent guidance about medicines and other treatment methods.

5. Voluntary Health Agencies

These groups collect money and information to fight various diseases. Some furnish treatment through their own centers. Others bring together people with various conditions so that they may profit from sharing their experiences. The American Cancer Society is the largest voluntary health agency.

6. Consumer Publications

Most prominent of these is Consumers Union, publisher of *Consumer Reports* and special publications. *Consumer Reports* has a circulation of two million. It contains many extremely well-written articles about health. Many of these have been compiled into *The Medicine Show*. This book evaluates over-the-counter drugs and health supplies in order to help you avoid wasting your money on products which don't work. Your library probably carries the publications of Consumers Union.

Now let's suppose you have a health problem or question. Where do you go? The best source is probably your own doctor. Chapters 5 and 24 of this book should help you find a doctor you can trust. If he can't answer your need, he should be able to help you find the answer.

What if he can't? Or what if you want to get reading material or general information? There are many places you can contact. If you write for information, be sure to keep in mind that the person who receives your letter may be extremely busy. You will most likely get a helpful response if you do the following:

1. Type your letter.
2. Ask your question in as specific a way as possible.
3. Tell something about yourself and why you need the information. Indicate what you already know or have read (briefly).
4. Enclose a large enough stamped, self-addressed envelope.
5. Consider making a small donation if you can afford one.

Here are the names of organizations which offer reliable health information and sometimes free services. Most of them are non-profit and non-commercial. Use them in good health!

Action on Smoking and Health, 2000 H Street, N.W., Washington, D.C. 20006

Aging Research Institute, 342 Madison Avenue, New York, N.Y. 10017

Alcohol, Drug Abuse and Mental Health Administration, U.S. Dept. of Health, Education and Welfare, 5600 Fishers Lane, Rockville, Md. 20852

Alcoholics Anonymous, P. O. Box 459, New York, N.Y. 10017

Alexander Graham Bell Association for the Deaf, 3417 Volta Place, N.W., Washington, D.C. 20007

Allergy Foundation of America, 801 Second Avenue, New York, N.Y. 10017

American Academy of Family Physicians, 1740 W. 92nd Street, Kansas City, Mo. 64114

American Academy of Pediatrics, 1801 Hinman Avenue, Evanston, Illinois 60204

American Alliance for Health, Physical Education and Recreation, 1201 16th Street, N.W., Washington, D.C. 20036

American Association on Mental Deficiency, 5201 Connecticut Avenue, N.W., Washington, D.C. 20015

American Cancer Society, 777 Third Avenue, New York, N.Y. 10017

American Cleft Palate Association, University of North Carolina School of Dentistry, Chapel Hill, N.C. 27514

American College of Sports Medicine, 1440 Monroe Street, Madison, Wis. 53706

American Dental Association, 211 E. Chicago Avenue, Chicago, Ill. 60611

American Diabetes Association, 1 W. 48th Street, New York, N.Y. 10020

American Dietetic Association, 430 N. Michigan Avenue, Chicago, Ill. 60611

American Foundation for the Blind, 15 W. 16th Street, New York, N.Y. 10011

American Geriatrics Society, 10 Columbus Circle, New York, N.Y. 10019

American Heart Association, 44 E. 23rd Street, New York, N.Y. 10010

American Hospital Association, 840 N. Lake Shore Drive, Chicago, Ill. 60611

American Lung Association (formerly National Tuberculosis and Respiratory Disease Association), 1740 Broadway, New York, N.Y. 10019

American Medical Association, 535 N. Dearborn Street, Chicago, Ill. 60610

American Medical Women's Association, 1740 Broadway, New York, N.Y. 10019

American Medical Writers Association, 9650 Rockville Pike, Bethesda, Md. 20014

American Nurses Association, 2420 Pershing Road, Kansas City, Mo. 64108

American Nursing Home Association, 1200 15th Street, N.W., Washington, D.C. 20005

American Occupational Therapy Association, 6000 Executive Blvd., Rockville, Md. 20852

American Optometric Association, 7000 Chippewa Street, St. Louis, Mo. 63119

American Osteopathic Association, 212 E. Ohio Street, Chicago, Illinois 60611

American Pharmaceutical Association, 2215 Constitution Avenue, N.W., Washington, D.C. 20037

American Physical Therapy Association, 1156 15th Street, N.W., Washington, D.C. 20005

American Podiatry Association, 20 Chevy Chase Circle, N.W., Washington, D.C. 20005

American Psychiatric Association, 1700 18th Street, N.W., Washington, D.C. 20009

American Psychoanalytic Association, One E. 57th Street, New York, N.Y. 10022

American Psychological Association, 1200 17th Street, N.W., Washington, D.C. 20036

American Public Health Association, 1015 18th Street, N.W., Washington, D.C. 20036

American Red Cross, 17th and D Streets, N.W., Washington, D.C. 20006

American Rehabilitation Foundation, 1800 Chicago Avenue, Minneapolis, Minn. 55404

American Social Health Association (venereal disease), 1740 Broadway, New York, N.Y. 10019

American Society of Clinical Hypnosis, 2400 E. Devon Avenue, Des Plains, Ill. 60018

American Speech and Hearing Association, 9030 Old Georgetown Road, Bethesda, Md. 20014

Arthritis Foundation, 475 Riverside Drive, New York, N.Y. 10027

Association for the Advancement of Health Education, 1201 16th Street, N.W., Washington, D.C. 20036

Association for Sickle Cell Anemia, 521 Fifth Avenue, New York, N.Y. 10036

Association for the Study of Abortion, 120 W. 57th Street, New York, N.Y. 10019

Better Vision Institute, 230 Park Avenue, New York, N.Y. 10017

Blue Cross Association, 842 N. Lake Shore Drive, Chicago, Ill. 60611

Braille Institute of America, 741 N. Vermont Avenue, Los Angeles, Calif. 90029

Cancer Care, Inc., One Park Avenue, New York, N.Y. 10016

Consumers Union, 256 Washington Street, Mt. Vernon, N.Y. 10550

Cooley's Anemia Foundation, 3366 Hillside Avenue, New Hyde Park, N.Y. 10040

Deafness Research Foundation, 366 Madison Avenue, New York, N.Y. 10017

Drug Abuse Council, 1828 L Street, N.W., Washington, D.C. 20036

Epilepsy Foundation of America, 1828 L Street, N.W., Washington, D.C. 20036

Euthanasia Educational Council, 250 W. 57th Street, New York, N.Y. 10019

Family Health (a publication), 545 Madison Avenue, New York, N.Y. 10022

Family Service Association of America, 44 E. 23rd Street, New York, N.Y. 10010

Gambler's Anonymous, P. O. Box 17173, Los Angeles, Calif. 90017

Health Education Council, 92 Belmont Drive, Livingston, N.J. 07039

Institute for Rehabilitation Medicine, 400 E. 34th Street, New York, N.Y. 10016

Institute for Sex Research, Inc., Indiana University, Bloomington, Ind. 47401

International Association of Laryngectomies, c/o American Cancer Society, 777 Third Avenue, New York, N.Y. 10017

Jewish Guild for the Blind, 15 W. 65th Street, New York, N.Y. 10023

Little People of America (dwarfism), Box 126, Owatonna, Minn. 55060

Maternity Center Association, 48 E. 92nd Street, New York, N.Y. 10028

Medical Library Association, 919 N. Michigan Avenue, Chicago, Illinois 60611

Muscular Dystrophy Associations of America, 810 Seventh Avenue, New York, N.Y. 10019

Myasthenia Gravis Foundation, 230 Park Avenue, New York, N.Y. 10017

National Family Planning Council, 1800 N. Highland Avenue, Los Angeles, Calif. 90028

National Amputation Foundation, 12–45 150th Street, Whitestone, N.Y. 11357

National Association of Blue Shield Plans, 211 E. Chicago Avenue, Chicago, Ill. 60611

National Association of Hearing and Speech Agencies, 814 Thayer Avenue, Silver Springs, Md. 20910

National Association for Mental Health, 1800 N. Kent Street, Arlington, Va. 22209

National Association for Retarded Citizens, P. O. Box 6109, Arlington, Texas, 76011

National Association of Social Workers, 1425 H Street, N.W., Washington, D.C. 20005

National Clearinghouse for Drug Abuse Information, 5600 Fishers Lane, Rockville, Md. 20852

National Council on Alcoholism, Two Park Avenue, New York, N.Y. 10016

National Cystic Fibrosis Foundation, 3379 Peach Tree Road, N.E., Atlanta, Ga. 30326

National Easter Seal Society for Crippled Children and Adults, 2023 W. Ogden Avenue, Chicago, Ill. 60612

National Foundation for Ileitis and Colitis, 295 Madison Avenue, New York, N.Y. 10017

National Foundation/March of Dimes, Box 2000, White Plains, N.Y. 10602

National Foundation for Sudden Infant Death, 1501 Broadway, New York, N.Y. 10036

National Genetics Foundation, 250 W. 57th Street, New York, N.Y. 10019

National Health Council, 1740 Broadway, New York, N.Y. 10019

National Hemophilia Foundation, 25 W. 39th Street, New York, N.Y. 10018

National Institute of Mental Health, 5600 Fishers Lane, Rockville, Md. 20852

National Interagency Council on Smoking and Health, 419 Park Avenue S., New York, N.Y. 10016

National Kidney Foundation, 116 E. 27th Street, New York, N.Y. 10016

National League for Nursing, 10 Columbus Circle, New York, N.Y. 10019

National Multiple Sclerosis Society, 257 Park Avenue S., New York, N.Y. 10010

National Nutrition Consortium, 9650 Rockville Pike, Bethesda, Md. 20014

National Nutrition Exchange, 55 Union Street, San Francisco, Calif. 94111

National Paraplegia Foundation, 333 N. Michigan Avenue, Chicago, Illinois 60601

National Parkinson Foundation, 1501 N.W. Ninth Avenue, Miami, Fla. 33136

National Public Relations Council of Health and Welfare Services, 815 Second Avenue, New York, N.Y. 10017

National Rehabilitation Association, 1522 K Street, N.W., Washington, D.C.   20005

National Society of Autistic Children, 169 Tampa Avenue, Albany, N.Y.   12208

National Safety Council, 425 N. Michigan Avenue, Chicago, Illinois   60611

National Society for the Prevention of Blindness, 79 Madison Avenue, New York, N.Y.   10016

National Student Nurses Association, 10 Columbus Circle, New York, N.Y.   10019

National Tay-Sachs and Allied Diseases Association, 122 E. 42nd Street, New York, N.Y.   10017

National Wheelchair Athletic Association, 40–24 62nd Street, Woodside, N.Y.   11377

Nutrition Foundation, 489 Fifth Avenue, New York, N.Y.   10017

Patients Aid Society, 509 Fifth Avenue, New York, N.Y.   10017

Planned Parenthood/World Population, 515 Madison Avenue, New York, N.Y.   10022

Seeing Eye (dogs for the blind), Washington Valley Road, Morristown, N.J.   07960

Suicide Prevention Center of Los Angeles, 1041 Menlo Avenue, Los Angeles, Calif.   90006

United Cerebral Palsy Associations, 66 E. 34th Street, New York, N.Y.   10016

United Ostomy Association, 1111 Wilshire Blvd., Los Angeles, Calif.   90017

20

QUACKERY AND THE MEDIA

A climate of hope and fear.

BY

MAX GUNTHER

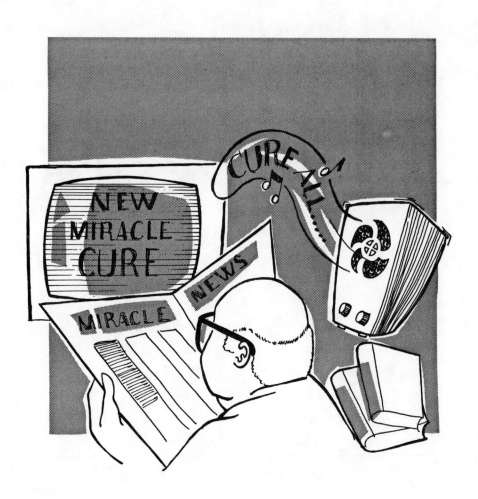

In an eventful quarter-century of writing for *Time* Magazine and as a freelancer, I've learned much about the internal mechanisms of "the media" as a message market place. The media have four main functions: to entertain, to inform, to carry advertisements, and to make money for their stockholders. Because of the ways in which these functions are carried out, and the peculiar and intricate ways in which they are connected, an appalling amount of misinformation— ranging from the faintly biased to the downright wrong—is fed every day to an unfortunately gullible public. Hardly anywhere is this more evident than in the fields of medicine and its unwanted cousin, medical quackery.

It is easy for those not in the print or TV or radio journalism business to decry this admittedly sorry state of affairs. It is easy to mount a podium and say, "The media should tell us the truth!" Easy to say, but not to translate into action.

Let Me Tell You a Story

Late in the 1960s a national women's magazine asked me to write an article about "beauty quackery." I was to cover such topics as inept nose-bobbing, face-peeling by nonprofessionals, fake vitality nostrums, and so on. In the course of the article I made some unenthusiastic remarks about a then-popular reducing machine sold under the trade name Relax-A-Cisor. It was supposed to trim bulging bodies by giving its users little electric shocks to induce muscle contractions which were alleged to produce the same results as healthy exercise. It didn't work (except for some people as a bizarre sexual stimulant), and even as I was writing the article, various government agencies were trying to drive it off the market. It has since been banned.

The magazine's nonfiction editor liked the article ex-

285

cept for one passage. Would I mind, the editor asked, if she were to cut out the reference to Relax-A-Cisor? The reason she gave was straightforward and practical. Relax-A-Cisor regularly bought advertising space in the magazine.

Well, what could I say? It would be naive to expect that a magazine, dependent on advertisers for its very life, would want to make a good advertiser mad. I told the editor I was more a practical journalist than an idealist and hence could sympathize with her problem. She and I agreed that this isn't the best of all possible worlds and that compromises, even unpleasant ones, are often necessary. I said, "Okay, kill the reference to your beloved advertiser." But I also said, "Please leave in the rest of my comments." These comments were to the effect that some electric reducing machines can be dangerous and that no machine can reduce weight all by itself.

A compromise. Not entirely satisfactory—but I went away with a shrug.

Then I saw the story in galley proof. By then I had reached a stage in my life when I thought nothing that happened in the media could shock me any more, but this did.

The editor and her colleagues had added a clever little embellishment to my words. They had written in some extra sentences that said, in effect: Sure, some reducing machines have been discredited. But, they added: "Most of those still being sold are legitimate. Used faithfully they *do* take off inches."

Unquote. A piece of gratuitous bootlicking, and moreover an outright lie. I grabbed the phone in a rage. The editor blamed the advertising sales director, who in turn blamed the corporate lawyers. "Look, we can't be printing nasty stuff about our advertisers," said the ad chief. I conceded that point. I had already conceded it to the editor. "But listen," I said, "you did more than just avoid making these people mad. You went out of your way to give a worthless gadget a free plug. You printed a plain, old-fashioned, damned lie under my name." The ad man finally said, "Well, yeah, maybe we did go overboard a bit, but—"

But what? But this is the way the media world works. What we want isn't always what we get. We start out wishing to tell the truth—and I believe that magazine editor started with such a wish in her heart—but then circumstances get in the way.

The Fear

Fear of losing good advertisers is one of the more common reasons why worthless medicines and gadgets and treatment methods get free plugs, and why you don't see honest medical rebuttals printed or aired as often as could be wished. A physician and professor at Northwestern University's School of Medicine, for example, is writing a book right now on a new, drug-free approach to headache treatment that he has developed and studiously tested. In this book he offers evidence that many common, over-the-counter headache remedies are potentially hazardous. Will he ever get to publicize this book by appearing on a TV talk show? Will any major magazine print a pre-publication excerpt? Both these questions make him gloomy.

"No TV station is going to let me stand up and advise people not to take pills for headaches," he says. "Nor will any of the big newsstand magazines. They all get lots of income from pill companies."

It seems significant that the hardest-hitting anti-quackery articles always appear in publications that don't make money from quacks of the given breed. For example, *Consumer Reports* has printed many articles attacking vitamin quackery and other nostrums. *Consumer Reports* carries no advertising at all. "For us," says senior editor Joseph Botta, "it's easier than for a lot of others. We never have ad backlash to worry about. Lots of other kinds of backlash, yes—but ad backlash is one worry we escape."

Let's look at those other kinds of backlash. Editor Botta is referring particularly to the kind that arises when people you attack are organized into a powerful and purposeful group. Chiropractors, for example. Botta's magazine ran a two-part report on chiropractic in 1975. The report wasn't an all-out attack, but its general conclusions were not encouraging.

"We got hundreds of letters," Botta recalls. "Chiropractors do a lot of letter-writing. When they're mad at somebody, their publications give the somebody's address and urge all the readers to bury the offender in mail. Well, we got buried. The letters said we were biased, inaccurate, in the employ of the AMA. 'How much did the AMA pay you?' some of them asked."

Ann Landers, the newspaper personal-advice columnist, had a similar experience. "I've taken on chiropractors periodically since I began writing the column 22 years ago," she says. "The last time was two years ago, and right away the chiropractors printed my address in their journals and told everybody to write. What I got was about 17,000 letters."

It is unpleasant for any writer or editor to receive all that nasty mail, but the mere anticipation of being buried in disagreeable letters doesn't generally keep anti-quackery material from being printed or broadcast. What more powerfully deters a journalist is fear of the economic or legal reprisals that such letters often threaten.

Joseph Botta, who has studied this matter from his

enviable position on a magazine independent of advertising, reports that less fortunate editors can be panicked by such threats. If a fringe pseudo-medical group discovers in advance that an unfavorable report on its activities is being prepared for publication or broadcast, he says, dark hints and warnings begin to flow through the mail. "They threaten to go to the advertisers and say, 'This publication or this TV station is about to run some libelous accusations against us. We suggest you withdraw your support. If you don't, we'll organize a boycott of your product.' An advertiser hates to hear talk of boycotts, even on a relatively small scale. Boycotts bring messy public relations problems he can do without. So he goes to the publication or the station and says, 'Look, I don't want to bring economic pressure to bear on you guys, but do you really *have* to run this quackery report?' " After the editor or producer has received similar gentle inquiries from several more advertisers, he begins to think that maybe the quackery report isn't such a good idea after all.

Threats of legal action are also scary, though for different reasons. "What troubles you isn't usually the fear of losing a lawsuit," said David Murray, who was editor of the consumer magazine, *Today's Health*, when the AMA stopped publishing it in 1976. "If we're going to publish a story that makes unkind statements about any health group, we go to great lengths to make sure our facts are well-documented, and we have our lawyers comb the piece for potential libel and other legal problems. We've been sued and threatened with suits by all kinds of groups, but we always feel pretty confident about our defense. The thing that troubles us is the enormous amount of time and work that one of these legal battles involves. Even when you win, you lose."

The fear of this losing-though-winning effect is something that keeps many potentially valuable anti-quack books and articles from ever being written. Shortly after *TV Guide* printed an article of mine on diet clap-trap, a New York publisher approached me with the suggestion that I write a "really honest, hard-hitting" book on the topic. I was attracted to the notion because, in researching and writing the article, I had become deeply concerned about the amount of food nonsense being swallowed by the unsuspecting public. Besides, I thought the project might be fun. I went around to see the chief editor, and he took me to lunch in one of those dim, expensive little restaurants where New York book people like to squander their expense accounts.

Over a pre-lunch martini, I told him of my private nightmare. "The kind of book you want," I said, "is the kind of book that could get us into libel suits. I'd need a lot of protection from you."

"Sure," he said. "That's understood."

"Well, but every book contract I've ever signed has had a legal escape clause for the publisher. Your contracts probably have one too, and that worries me."

The escape clauses to which I was referring are standard on all book contracts. A typical one now lying on my desk says: "The Author represents, warrants and covenants that the Work . . . contains no libelous or other unlawful matter . . . The Author agrees to indemnify and hold harmless the Publisher . . . against loss or expense, including court costs and attorneys' fees . . ."

In other words, the poor old Author is on his own if he annoys a quack and the quack sues. My editor friend acknowledged that there was such a clause in his company's standard contract. "But look," he said, "in prac-

290

tice those clauses are pretty well ignored. Most publishers will back up an author if he gets hauled into court, and we'll back you up."

"That's nice," I said, "but I think I'd feel more comfortable if you struck out the escape clause altogether. Will you?"

"I'll see what can be done," he said dubiously.

"Also," I said, "the biggest worry I have isn't about losing a lawsuit. It's about losing time and earnings. Suppose one of these cases drags on for months. Suppose I have to spend a lot of time talking to lawyers, sitting around in courtrooms, digging out research material to shore up my defense. Would you help me out?"

"Well," he said, still more dubiously, "I guess we could always arrange some kind of advance against future royalties, or something."

"In other words lend me my own money," I said. "That wasn't what I meant. Look, if *you* have to spend time on a lawsuit arising from one of your books, the company goes on paying your salary, right? But I'm a freelancer. When I don't work at my profession, I don't get paid. *That*'s my big nightmare."

"Well, what are you asking me to do?"

"Share the risk with me. You want me to write a tough book about quacks, and the quacks are going to get mad, and I don't want to take the punishment all alone. So I'm asking you to put a risk-sharing clause in the contract. If some quack files suit and I get taken away from my typewriter, your company pays me a daily living allowance until we're out of the soup."

He leaned back in his chair, heaved a big sigh and finally said, softly, "Oh boy."

And so an anti-quackery book, which might have been a useful one, never got written. There is no way of knowing how many other quack-exposing books and magazine articles and TV shows have died in the womb for similar reasons, but I am certain the number is large.

Even when a writer and editor do get together and swallow their fears and decide to produce a forthright report, they may be hampered by the fact that legitimate medical scientists harbor the same fears. If I were to have written that book on diet quackery, I would have needed to find serious nutritionists and other authorities who were willing to talk to me, to be quoted by name, and to make anti-quack statements in plain English. But physicians, like writers and everybody else, are reluctant to be dragged into unpleasant, time-consuming squabbles. I might have found too few brave men and women to make a book.

The Open Door Policy

Those are some of the reasons why relatively few critical reports on fringe medical practices are printed or broadcast. Now let's look at the problem from the opposite direction. Why do the media give so much free space and air time to proponents of bizarre health theories?

On TV, the Merv Griffin Show is notorious as an electronic soapbox for health nuts. If you want to get yourself interviewed on that show, all that seems to be required is that you invent some weird new medical or medical-mystical idea, that you write a book or gather some kind of following behind you, and that you and your idea be colorful. Two requirements that decidedly don't exist are that your medical views have a sound basis in recognizable science or that they be endorsed or at least considered plausible by the AMA.

When medical scientists challenge Griffin about this, he and his colleagues give answers that cannot be ar-

gued with. Not easily, anyhow. William Barron, publicity spokesman for the show, points out piously but with
justification that our society guarantees a hearing to
the iconoclast, the challenger of established views,
even the madman. "This show has an open-door policy," Barron says. "If somebody has something interesting to say, this is one place where he can say it
without being heckled."

That is perfectly proper, of course. It would not be in
America's best interests to close that or other doors. You
and I have the right to say what we want to say, even if
our words anger other people.

Barron insists further, in the Griffin show's defense,
that its approach is "reportorial, non-judgmental." But
Griffin seldom invites qualified medical scientists onto
his stage to rebut the peculiar notions that have been
left drifting around. Many worried men and women
have asked for equal time, and some have been given it
but most haven't. The National Nutrition Consortium,
for example, asked for time to rebut a presentation on
the supposed healthful effects of massive vitamin
doses. The group wanted to tell the scientific side of the
story: that there is little evidence that such big doses
can do you much good, while there is evidence of potentially dangerous toxic effects. A year after sending its
letter requesting equal time, the Consortium still
hadn't received a reply.

Why not? Undoubtedly part of the answer, if not the
whole of it, is that the show's producers felt the proposed rebuttal would be much less interesting than the
original presentation. "People with bizarre medical
theories are often very colorful, very entertaining," remarks Dr. Philip L. White, chief public spokesman of
the AMA Council on Foods and Nutrition. "Obviously,
any TV talk show wants colorful and entertaining
guests. We scientific types, by contrast, are pretty dull

clods. We always find ourselves in the position of prick-
ing people's balloons. We're always having to say, 'No,
this quick and magical cure won't work.' "

Dr. White is so convinced of his own dullness (though
in fact he is an uncommonly witty fellow!) that he
never asks for TV or radio rebuttal time and studiously
avoids those one-to-one confrontations in which a recognized authority and a health faddist hold an on-
the-air debate. He has morosely watched many
such debates, he says, and has never seen one in
which the scientific man came out ahead. "The anti-
establishment man is almost always the more flam-
boyant and interesting, almost always has glib, quick,
confident answers ready. The scientific rebuttals are
usually dry, unemotional, complex, hard to explain or
understand—for that is the very nature of science, isn't
it? It's a fight that can't be won in a half-hour TV
show."

Not only are off-trail health ideas colorful, but they
sell. This is another reason why they command so much
media space and time. They offer the "quick" and
"magical" results that Dr. White mentions, so people
rush to buy them. *Dr. Atkins' Diet Revolution*, for instance, is a how-to-get-slim book whose rationale the
AMA Council finds "for the most part without scientific
merit." Yet more than a million copies were sold in the
first year after its publication—a record for any
hardcover book of any kind. Why? Because it offered
what sounded like a quick, easy way to shed fat. *It
offered magic.*

Another slimming plan that sounded magical, but
that scientists regarded without enthusiasm, was published in 1974 by *Family Circle* magazine. The plan
was grandly titled, "My Amazing Cider Vinegar,
Lecithin, Kelp, B_6 Diet." It consisted of adding the four
ingredients listed in the title to a low-calorie diet. This

294

"mysterious mixture," suggested the author Mary Ann Crenshaw, made the diet "seemingly infallible for making *my* weight come off in a sudden rush."

But Dr. White and other nutrition scientists, dull clods that they are, insist that the *only* thing which determines weight loss is taking in fewer calories than your body expends. Each 3,500 calorie deficit will lose you a pound and that's that. No exotic foodstuff (such as kelp, a seaweed whose taste reminds me of wet newspaper) will increase the speed with which your fat disappears.

Family Circle readers evidently hoped otherwise. The magazine's space sales department, in an effort to lure more advertisers to the magazine, bragged later that readers had "emptied the shelves" of kelp and that other stuff. Why the buying rush? Again, an offer of magic.

I sent my research associate around to ask *Family Circle* some questions about all this. We wanted to know if the magazine had tested the diet before publishing it, if the editors had sought independent medical opinions, and so on. Health Editor Maxine Lewis, noting with a chuckle that the subject was "touchy," amiably but firmly declined to talk to us unless we submitted a list of questions in advance. Foreseeing delays, we abandoned the probe.

Now let's ask if anything can be done to attack all these problems. There do seem to be two possibilities:

A Countervailing Push

One of journalism's major problems in this field is that there is very little *push* in the direction of sound, carefully researched medical reporting. There are three possible approaches that a writer or editor or TV producer can take toward a given brand of quackery: he can be friendly to it, he can ignore it, or he can attack it. Of the three, the last is vastly the hardest.

Consider the legal push. There are libel laws to make us nervous when we attack anybody in the media. These laws are reasonably clearcut. Their teeth may not be as long or sharp as some media people fear, but when you see a shark in the water, it makes you careful. The libel laws represent a clearly felt danger. On the other hand, there is no countervailing body of law to make us careful when we give public praise to quacks, and of course there is no law against ignoring them either.

Suppose I write, "Dr. Schrunkenkopf's Magic Sex-Regeneration and Dandruff Pills are nothing but sugar, and Schrunkenkopf is a quack." I write myself into trouble. If I am determined to write it, I must do a lot of hard work to make sure that what I say is soundly documented. On the other hand, with no research at all and with no feeling of danger I can write, "Dr. Schrunkenkopf is a great healer and scholar, and a lot of people say his amazing pills have cured their sex problems and dandruff, and furthermore the pills taste terrific!" Or, choosing the middle course and ignoring the issue, I can write simply, "Dr. Schrunkenkopf announced that his Magic Sex-Regeneration and Dandruff Pills will henceforth be offered in a choice of two colors." If I choose either of these easy courses, I know nobody will seriously attack me. I may receive a few grumpy letters from honest doctors and perhaps one from the AMA. These, of course, can be quietly filed in my wastebasket.

Or, let's suppose a book publisher approaches me tomorrow with a self-styled "doctor" in tow—and the doctor has rigged up a sensational new diet that lets you stuff yourself with meat and cake, makes you thin, gives you hypnotic power over members of the opposite sex, prevents cancer, and cures athlete's foot. The publisher wants me to ghostwrite a book on this diet in collaboration with the doctor. He informs me that the advance bidding from paperback companies is already approaching a million dollars, and so is the European bidding, and my earnings are guaranteed to be at least $250,000. What answer do I give? What should I do?

Ah, what indeed? All the push is in the wrong direction. The only thing standing in the way of this push, absolutely the only obstacle, is my own frail conscience!

I don't really know what I would do. But I suspect, in the end, my conscience would buckle.

What is needed is a countervailing push. There should be some kind of punishment for writing favorably about quackery, something to make the easy course less easy, some clearly perceived danger.

What might this be? Pressure from peer-review boards has sometimes been suggested. At present the two most prominent groups in the journalistic peer-review business are Accuracy In Media (AIM) and the National News Council (NNC). Such outfits, however, lack force. The most they can do, essentially, is grumble at people. Moreover, it is obvious that they can devote only a minor share of their time to the specific problem of medical quackery. There are too many other media problems to worry about.

Thus, it would seem, the countervailing pressure against quackery in the media must come from the medical world, not the journalistic world. It must come from some group that is concerned with this specific media problem to the exclusion of others. The group's first order of business should be to explore this problem of incentive.

Somehow, the countervailing push must be made

more forceful than it has ever been in the past. Perhaps the question could be explored in cooperation with government agencies or legal groups. The point will be to create a situation in which it is as risky to give favorable exposure to Schrunkenkopf's Pills as to damn them.

An Ammunition Depot

Another reason why dubious health ideas get a lot of favorable coverage is that media folk, like everybody else, tend to be lazy. If I start out with no particular bias for or against a given issue, I will often casually adopt the bias contained in whatever material comes easily to hand. Quacks and health nuts, as a breed, are well aware of this and usually stand ready to hand any inquiring reporter a fat, juicy dossier of misinformation promoting their views. If the reporter is conscientious enough to seek a scientific medical opinion on that dossier, his search may go unrewarded. He may find a couple of doctors who are willing to give him the facts—"but for God's sake don't quote me by name." Or he may find nobody at all. In the end he gives up and simply writes what the dossier says.

Anti-fluoridation forces in many communities have used this phenomenon to great advantage. It is very easy to write a sensational story on the dangers of fluoride-treated water. All a reporter need do is go to the local anti-fluoride group, and the group will hand him a thick file of horrible case histories, ghastly statistics, and so on. The group, in effect, hands him his story on a silver tray. Seldom will he find a responsible medical or dental group in the community that has any such well-organized promotion campaign. Seldom will his pro-fluoride file grow half as thick or as deliciously scary as the other one. Most often, responsible medical opinion will be represented by a couple of doctors who say,

"Maybe, but on the other hand . . . and don't quote me!"

What medical science needs to do is to make good stories as easy to find as bad ones. Every county medical society ought to have a well-publicized phone number that any reporter or TV producer can call for information on any health topic. When he calls that number, he ought to be referred to a physician or group of physicians who will give him solid information on his topic, straight answers in plain English—and who, just as important, will not only permit him to quote them by name but will invite him to do so. Their story, like the health faddists', ought to come to him on a silver tray.

As things are today, this kind of medical response happens all too seldom. The AMA has long been a source of anti-quackery ammunition and can do an excellent job of answering media folks' questions and referring them to knowledgeable specialists. However, the AMA headquarters and press office are in Chicago. Not many media people, particularly not many who work for local publications or broadcasting stations, ever bother to make the necessary phone call.

If there were local anti-quackery ammuntion depots as clever and efficient as AMA's national one, honest medical science would get its story told more fully in the media. Each depot should be set up to *welcome* media inquiries—something that has been rather rare in the past. What happens most often today, when you phone some local medical group or organization in search of a story, is that you are treated like a damned nuisance. A bored-voiced woman answers your call, listens without enthusiasm to what you want, says she will "check on it" and call you back. She doesn't call you back. You repeat the call and finally get a doctor on the phone. The doctor is either too busy to talk to you or too scared or both. You go away thinking, "Well,

Schrunkenkopf may be crazy, but at least he's quotable
. . ."

The medical world and the media world can surely learn to communicate better. It seems unlikely that quackery will ever be wiped out, but at least its voice can be muted.

21

THE FEDS

Many people believe that advertising claims must be true or else "they wouldn't be allowed." We wish that were so.

BY

IRENE L. BARTLETT
*Ex-Program Associate
American Cancer Society*

Early in 1972, a housewife complained to postal authorities about a "reducing pill" called "Slim-Tabs." Sold by mail, the pill cost from $5.98 for a 15-day supply to $15.00 for a 60-day supply. Customers were promised weight losses of up to 48 pounds in eight weeks. During the first half of 1972, promoters of Slim-Tabs did more than $1,000,000 worth of business.

In July 1972, however, two months after the postal investigation began, a New Jersey federal court gave permission for postal authorities to hold mail addressed to Slim-Tabs' promoters while further legal steps were taken. Early in 1973, some 58,000 letters were returned to their senders and three of Slim-Tabs' principal promoters pleaded guilty to mail fraud charges.

Though its dollar amount is higher than the usual, this case illustrates the work of the U.S. Postal Inspector in combatting quackery. The Postal Service has jurisdiction over any case which uses the mail to transfer money in payment for products or services. Five full-time inspectors work in a special division which handles health frauds. They are assisted by eight more liaison inspectors who are stationed in large cities. Additional help is available from inspectors who usually work on other matters.

Health frauds come to the attention of postal inspectors in several ways. Complaints are received from the general public, both directly and through Congressmen. Inspectors monitor ads in magazines, newspapers, and radio and television commercials. Complaints are also referred by other government agencies.

The aim of the postal inspector is to find out promptly whether false representations have been made and to stop illegal schemes before too many mail customers have been cheated or hurt. Investigation of a complaint is done in a variety of ways. Test letters may be sent by inspectors posing as customers. Sample products may be bought and analyzed by the FDA Chemical Analysis and Medical Laboratory—the largest and most modern facility in the world devoted to research on foods, drugs and cosmetics. From the thousands of complaints it receives each year, the Postal Service selects those which it feels are most significant—those which will generate a large amount of mail or which are the most dangerous to the public.

Prosecution

The United States Code provides the Postal Service with a variety of legal weapons against false representations. Title 39, Section 3005, can be used to prevent promoters of misleading schemes from receiving money or orders through the mail. While action under Section 3005 is under way, if sufficient health hazard exists, an immediate court order to impound mail may be sought under Section 3007 of the Code. This procedure can stop a dangerous operation very quickly, but it is used only in high priority cases—such as worthless cancer cures or a treatment for facial blemishes which removes the face also.

Title 18, Section 1341, provides for criminal prosecution. The maximum penalties are a fine of $1,000, five years in prison, or both. Under this section, intent to deceive must be proved—a task which can be difficult and time-consuming. Though Section 1341 is used sparingly, almost all cases actually brought to trial result in convictions.

Sometimes, when a promoter finds he is under investigation, he may decide to get out of business without further ado.

The FDA

The U.S. Food and Drug Administration has jurisdiction over labeling of foods, drugs, devices and cosmetics. Labeling is not limited to what is on a product's container. It also includes claims made in books, pamphlets, broadcasts, lectures or sales talks—as long as the claims are made in conjunction with sale of the product.

The FDA traces its roots to just after the turn of this century, when consumers needed all the protection they could get. Patent medicines which were worthless, but not always harmless, were widely promoted with cure-all claims. The country was plagued by unsanitary conditions in meat-packing plants. Harmful chemicals were being added to foods, and labels rarely told what their products contained.

The Pure Food and Drug Act, which was passed in 1906, has been strengthened by a number of amendments and related acts. Together, these various laws are concerned primarily with the accuracy and truthfulness of labeling. Under the 1938 Food, Drug and Cosmetic Act, false and misleading statements are banned from drug labels. Active ingredients must be listed, and products must be proven safe before marketing. Under the 1962 Kefauver-Harris Drug Amendments, products must be shown to be *effective* also.

FDA efforts to control health quackery are carried out mainly under three sections of the Food, Drug and Cosmetic Act. Section 502, parts (a), (f) and (j), defines misbranding. Section 301 defines prohibited acts and Section 303 describes penalties. Complaints are usually received from consumers, Congressmen, FDA field inspectors and various government agencies. Significant complaints are followed up by FDA field inspectors and evaluated by physicians and other scientists.

If investigation shows that a product is a "new drug," it must have FDA approval for movement in interstate commerce. Violation of this provision can lead to seizure and a court injunction. To be classified as a "new drug," a product does not actually have to be new. It could also be a familiar substance which has a new claim made for it. For example, a claim that wheat germ oil "prevents heart stress" would make the oil a new drug with respect to that particular claim.

Civil action will be taken in cases of minor violation. Criminal action is available for major ones. First offenders can be fined up to $1,000, imprisoned up to one year, or both. If an offense includes intent to defraud, however, the penalty can be as much as a $10,000 fine, three years in prison, or both.

The FTC

The Federal Trade Commission was established in 1914. Its original purpose was to safeguard businesses against monopoly and unfair competition. Five Commissioners who serve staggered terms head this agency. Control of health quackery was not a major concern of the early Commissioners. With the appointment of William E. Humphrey in 1925, however, there was a marked increase in the attack on false drug advertising. But until passage of the Wheeler-Lea Act in 1938, agency emphasis was on injury to competitors rather than consumers.

The FTC has jurisdiction over advertising of foods, non-prescription drugs, cosmetics and devices which are involved in interstate commerce. Section 12 of the Wheeler-Lea Act allows the government to attack false advertising which could injure consumers as well as competitors. In determining what is false, what is left out may be considered as well as what is said. If a problem is serious enough, a court injunction can halt the practice being challenged until the matter can be resolved under regular procedure.

The FTC has broad powers to investigate complaints. Uncooperative businessmen—who do not answer questions, reveal documents or respond to subpoena—are subject to heavy penalties. If investigation concludes that a law violation exists, the FTC will issue a Complaint. At this point, advertisers may comply voluntarily without admitting wrongdoing. If they resist, an Administrative Law Judge will hold a hearing which can lead to a "cease-and-desist" order. Such orders become final if not reviewed by the Commission. Commission decisions, in turn, are subject to appeal through federal courts.

Cease-and-desist orders set forth findings and prohibit respondents from engaging in alleged illegal practices. When final, these orders act as permanent injunctions. In 1972, the FTC reported that it was enforcing 7,500 of them. Penalties for violating consent agreements or cease-and-desist orders can be very heavy—including prison sentences and fines of up to $10,000 per day for continuing violations. Recently, for example, the J. B. Williams Company paid $302,000 as a result of violating cease-and-desist orders which prohibited various claims for *Geritol* and *FemIron*, two of its patent medicines.

In addition to cease-and-desist orders, the FTC issues industry guides and trade regulation rules. Guides are interpretive statements without the force of law. Rules represent the conclusions of the Commission about what it considers unlawful. Once a rule is established, lengthy explanations of the reasons why a particular ad is unfair or deceptive are no longer necessary. A reference to the rule is enough. Before guides and rules are established, interested parties are given the opportunity to comment.

Few guidelines have been issued in the area of health quackery, but several are now under consideration. An industry guide on food advertising, which included "health" and "organic" foods, was issued in 1974. In

1975, guidelines were proposed for testimonial advertising and for protein supplements (which are commonly promoted with misleading claims).

In 1972, the FTC began an Advertising Substantiation Program, under which it may require advertisers to prove claims of safety, performance, efficacy and comparative price. When information is received, it is made public so that consumers can evaluate the evidence for themselves. So far, relatively few of the advertising substantiations have been in the health field.

Effectiveness

Many people believe that claims for health products must be true or else "they wouldn't be allowed." We wish that were so. Spokesmen for each of the above agencies told me they felt they had good laws. But it is important to understand the limitations of these laws.

Federal agencies do not have the manpower to handle all cases which are reported to them, so they must assign priorities. As a result, some fraudulent promoters escape prosecution or are lightly punished.

Before legal action can be taken to control a fraud, it must be detected and then investigated. In many cases, rapid protection of the public is possible. The FDA can quickly ban use of an unapproved "new drug" in interstate commerce. The Postal Service may quickly block receipt of money obtained through the mail by fraud. But some promoters make considerable profit before their schemes are detected.

Each agency has problems related to the construction of its laws. The Postal Service has difficulty with promoters who, after settling one case of deceptive practice, begin a new one—hoping to profit before being stopped again. Repeat offenders, of course, are more likely to encounter criminal prosecution.

The main problem of the FTC is delay. Its internal procedures can take years to complete, and their effect can be postponed further by appeals through federal courts. In one celebrated case, it took the FTC 16 years to remove the word "Liver" from Carter's Little Liver Pills.

The FDA can also be hampered by court delay in major cases, but for the most part, its "new drug" regulation has driven false claims off product labels. Unfortunately, however, the health food industry is now able to sell its wares without making sales claims. The labels of products sold by the health food industry rarely tell why the products should be used. They don't have to—thanks to our media. News articles, books, magazine articles and radio and TV talk shows have done such a good sales job that everybody *knows* what food supplements are for.

You Can Help

The best protection against fraud is an informed consumer. All three of the above agencies can provide you with information about health frauds. If you have a question, or if a "health" promotion makes you suspicious, please contact the appropriate agency. If the product involves transfer of money through the mail, contact your local postal inspector or write directly to the Chief Postal Inspector, U.S. Postal Service, Washington, D.C. 20260. If a product label (or accompanying literature) contains questionable claims, it can be reported to your nearest FDA field office or to FDA headquarters at 5600 Fishers Lane, Rockville, Md. 20852. Suspicious advertising claims should be reported to the FTC Bureau of Consumer Protection, Washington, D.C. 20580.

In each instance, carefully note when and where you encountered the problem. Give the agency any suspicious advertisement or label. If an ad or product came by mail, include its wrapper. Tell the agency your name and address so that it can contact you if it needs further information.

Remember, the few minutes you take to report a fraud may save many people from being cheated—and might even save a life!

Recommended Reading

Fraud—The United States Postal Inspection Service and some of the fools and knaves it has known, by E. J. Kahn, Jr.

The Federal Trade Commission, by Susan Wagner.

The Medical Messiahs, by James Harvey Young.

22

PROGRESS IN PENNSYLVANIA

"Truth is always the strongest argument."
—Sophocles

BY

H. WILLIAM GROSS, D.D.S.
President, Lehigh Valley Committee
Against Health Fraud, Inc.

In December, 1969, a number of health professionals formed a small group to fight quackery. Local medical, dental, osteopathic, podiatric, optometric, pharmaceutical, nursing and health service organizations suggested additional members who were interested in this problem. An appeal to the local bar association brought several volunteer attorneys. By word of mouth, we attracted laymen with a variety of backgrounds—labor and industry leaders, teachers, ministers and homemakers.

At first we were sponsored by local professional societies. But we soon realized that a fast-moving, hard-hitting effort would require independence from them. So we incorporated as the Lehigh Valley Committee Against Health Fraud, Inc. Our financial support now comes mainly from individual contributions and sale of publications. With mostly volunteer labor, however, we don't need much money to be effective.

Currently, we have about 35 individual members whose interests, availability and talents are quite varied. Some are seasoned political activists, both in and out of the health field. Some are excellent writers and public speakers. Some have much time to give, others have little. All share a deep sense of fair play and interest in our fellow man. As time goes on, each of us carves out his or her own niche in our action network.

We do many things. We testify at various government hearings. We organize letter-writing campaigns when misinformation appears in newspapers or when pertinent legislation is being considered. We stimulate media coverage, providing accurate information and attacking misinformation and its promoters. We exchange ideas and publications with other groups and individuals. We furnish public speakers. We monitor publications and health food stores, reporting suspected violations to appropriate law enforcement agencies. During the past year alone, we sent about forty questionable ads for "health" products to the U.S. Postal Inspector's office. Most of these had appeared in *Moneysworth, Let's Live* magazine, *National Enquirer* and various chiropractic journals.

We also invite people who think they have been cheated in health matters to complain to us. In one such case (mentioned in Chapter 10), we helped three people recover $13,575 from a chiropractor who they claimed had cheated them. The chiropractor subsequently had his license suspended for six months. In another case, we helped an Allentown housewife collect $30,000 in an out-of-court settlement of a malpractice suit against an erring optometrist.

Groups like ours are badly needed to balance the enormous amount of misinformation that the public receives from radio and TV talk shows, advertisements, questionable publications and private conversations between promoters of quackery and their victims. In terms of impact, perhaps the worst offenders are TV talk shows which can reach very large audiences. Some of these promote serious misinformation on nutrition while offering little or no time for nutrition scientists to present accurate information. One group like ours has been formed in Quebec, Canada, under the leadership of Dr. Murray Katz. Another has been formed in Northern California and it looks as if a few others may get started in the near future. A national organization is badly needed to coordinate the activities and information-gathering of local groups and individuals. The AMA Department of Investigation used to do this to some extent, but it was abolished in 1975 when the AMA ran into financial difficulty.

In 1972, the Pennsylvania Health Council began a Committee on Health Fraud to expose deceptive health practices in Pennsylvania. Its initial plan was to conduct a series of regional conferences on health quackery to which the public would be invited. The first such program, which was held in Allentown in 1973, was a great success. More than 600 people visited its exhibits and the conference received a great deal of coverage in the news media. The second program, which took place in Pittsburgh a year later, was also a success. But unfortunately, the Pennsylvania Health Council encountered financial difficulty and has discontinued its health fraud committee.

In 1973, the Pennsylvania Medical Society formed a Committee on Quackery which now serves as a clearinghouse for complaints and inquiries from Pennsylvania physicians. Most state medical society quackery committees confine themselves to exposing chiropractic, but the PMS committee is concerned about all questionable health matters which come to its attention. In addition, the PMS committee has a unique source of operating funds. Known as the Quackery Defense Fund, it is supported by voluntary, annual $5 contributions from the Society's members. To date, the fund has received more than 10,000 individual donations.

Perhaps the PMS committee's most interesting project so far has been a series of public service messages which were distributed to radio stations throughout Pennsylvania. Each one was designed by the PMS communications division to counteract a widely-held myth about nutrition. Here's a sample:

(Sound of bottles being shuffled around)
Man: Honey, have you seen my pills?
Woman: You mean your vitamin E pills? Don't tell me you've been taking them again, Harry.
Man: (Embarrassed) You mean you haven't noticed? I mean, last night . . .

Woman: Harry, vitamin E doesn't help your
. . . uh . . . manly abilities.
Man: (Obviously embarrassed) But last
night . . . I thought . . .
Woman: What too much vitamin E can do is
give you headaches, nausea and muscle weakness. And, surprise . . . it
can actually reduce your sexual potency.
Man: But, last night.
Woman: (Firmly) I should know, Harry.

People sometimes ask how they might develop a group like ours in their own community. An excellent way to begin would be to form a reading group which meets once or twice a month. Each of the chapters of this book could be a subject for research and discussion. As your knowledge grows, form a speakers' bureau. Let the media and other community groups know you are available. As you study political forces and legislation affecting consumer protection in the field of health, you may wish to write letters to publications and legislators. Because people seldom take the trouble to do this, a group of individuals writing on a regular basis can make itself felt considerably out of proportion to its size.

Please feel free to contact us if you have any ideas, experiences or publications to share, questions to ask, projects to design or money to contribute. Our address is Box 1602, Allentown, Pa. 18105. If you share our deep interest, perhaps we can find ways to work together.

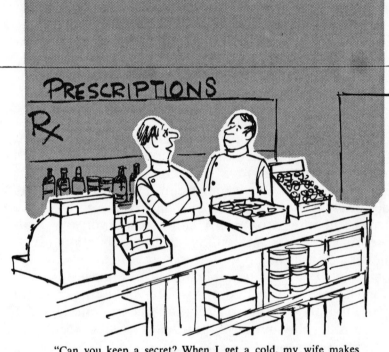

"Can you keep a secret? When I get a cold, my wife makes me tie an old sock with an onion in it around my neck."

WHY QUACKERY PERSISTS

While the physician seeks to help his patient if he can, he must sometimes confess that he cannot. The quack need make no such confession, for honesty is not contained in his code of ethics. This gives the charlatan great advantage in competing with the physician.

BY

JAMES HARVEY YOUNG, Ph.D.
Professor of History
Emory University

Americans have always been an optimistic people, have believed that problems are for solving. When quackery came to be recognized as a problem in the health field, many learned commentators predicted its certain death. Common sense, education, and the truths of science would drive quackery from the marketplace. Especially as modern medicine developed and conquered one disease after another, anything so outmoded and unneeded as quackery, some writers cheerfully suggested, would shortly wither away.

But this has not happened. Quite the contrary! Health quackery today is a multi-billion dollar business. Why does quackery persist so stubbornly in our modern scientific era? Let us seek an explanation for this curious fact by examining the roles of three parties involved—the patient, the orthodox practitioner, and the quack.

The Patient

The field of health is extremely complicated. John Doe, the common man, has absorbed a great mass of information about it. What he knows, however, is likely a jumble of chance facts learned from a variety of sources, sound and unsound, including the folklore of family tradition and the self-serving pitch of current advertising. Statistically, perhaps, most people may be nearer right than wrong, but few people escape blind spots and areas of error that make them vulnerable to deception under suitable circumstances. This goes for some John Does of mighty intellect with various degrees after their names.

When an episode of ill health looms, John Doe faces it either by self-reliance or by seeking help from a health authority. If he chooses self-treatment, he tries some remedy from folk tradition or from recent reading or television viewing. He may try garlic from the garden,

318

a huge dose of vitamin C, or a trade-named tonic. He tends to judge results by the same rule-of-thumb common sense by which he judges everyday cause-and-effect sequences: Did the axe cut? Did the suit fit? Did the motor run? He asks: Did the symptoms go away? Did my digestion settle down? Did my nerves calm? Did my sniffles stop?

John Doe does not usually realize that most ailments are self-limiting and improve with time *regardless of treatment*. When a symptom goes away after he doses himself with a remedy, he is likely to credit the remedy with curing him. He does not realize that he would have gotten better just as quickly if he had done nothing! Thousands of well-meaning John and Jane Does have boosted the fame of folk remedies and have signed sincere testimonials for patent medicines, crediting them instead of the body's recuperative powers for a return to well-being.

Nor does John Doe take the "placebo" effect into account when he judges remedies. Worry has a great effect upon how we feel when we are ill. The more we are worried about being sick, the more uncomfortable our symptoms will seem. Conversely, the less we are worried, the better we may feel. When John Doe takes a remedy that he thinks will help him, he will often feel less pain or discomfort. Feeling better when the doctor walks into the room is another example of this mechanism. The placebo effect can work in a second way. Some ailments which are body reactions to tension can subside when the feeling that a person is taking an effective treatment lessens the tension.

A considerable element of success of the legitimate proprietary remedies bought at the drugstore undoubtedly resides in the placebo effect. Spokesmen for the proprietary industry have occasionally acknowledged this. Exaggerated claims made in advertising may even build up the consumer's expectations and enlarge the placebo effect. Yet such a slim benefit does not justify exaggeration. Overuse of occasionally useful drugs poses health hazards. Youth's readiness to experiment with dangerous drugs may owe something to the attitude, conditioned by constant advertising, that a drug exists to banish almost any problem. A good deal of advertising implies that common remedies can somehow do more than relieve simple symptoms, can make a person socially desirable, can solve undesirable behavior like "snapping at your wife." Moreover, too much or too long reliance on self-dosage, in violation of label warnings, may lead people to delay getting more appropriate treatment for serious ailments before it is too late. Outright quackery, of course, operates without any of the restraints under which the proprietary industry abides and hence poses a danger greatly magnified.

The John Doe whom I have been describing so far turns to self-treatment occasionally when his normally healthy life is disrupted. Some of his unhappy cousins, however, live in constant fear of imminent health disaster. They seem governed by an all-consuming anxiety that leads to continuous self-treatment, often with bizarre "preventive" programs. An example might be taking 25 food supplement pills per day. Some beleaguered patients go so far as to follow all-inclusive systems which mix diet practices, exercises, gadgetry, and mystical philosophies. These troubled people, although a minority of the population, provide an important reservoir for quack exploitation.

Often, of course, such worriers abandon self-treatment and join a guru-led group—just as less extreme John and Jane Does might give up self-reliance and seek help from some authority. A great deal of public confusion exists about who is a competent health authority. In a medical world so full of specialists,

320

many people mistakenly think of chiropractors as specialists who treat back problems.

Some patients have an authority problem and tend to reject the orthodox merely because it is the orthodox. Other patients turn to unscientific practitioners under the miss-no-bets philosophy. They believe in family doctors as treaters of organic ailments and prescribers of drugs. They also believe in chiropractors as manipulators of bones and perhaps as operators of "healing" machines. They likewise follow the gospel of food faddists. And they sense nothing wrong with using several such forms of treatment at the same time, science and pseudoscience having equal importance in their minds.

One last point about the patient: When his health is seriously threatened, he obviously hopes something may be done to cure him. His desires may outrun what responsible orthodoxy can accomplish. Confronted with the possibility of chronic suffering or death, many people who never before strayed from orthodox treatment are not able to accept orthodoxy's grim verdict and so turn elsewhere. Such desperation has fattened cancer quackery.

The Orthodox Practitioner

The medical profession has always believed its current knowledge valid and has sometimes exhibited a tendency toward smugness. On occasion, true scientific breakthroughs may have been regarded as quackery. Conversely, many treatments which were once highly regarded have been abandoned as worthless. As medical science improves, of course, it becomes easier to draw the line between orthodoxy and quackery. Ignoring this fact, quacks parade medicine's old mistakes and portray themselves as scientists ahead of their time who are being suppressed by a greedy establishment.

321

Many people have suffered side effects from modern "miracle" drugs. This circumstance, added to the over-prescribing of antibiotics, tranquilizers, and stimulants, has helped foster a stereotype of our nation being "drugged," thereby giving "natural" healers a promotional boost. In the early 19th century, quacks termed the doctor a butcher. Today they call him a poisoner.

Orthodox physicians, moreover, have a problem because of their power and status. Non-experts feel ill at ease in the presence of an expert. The patient is upset because he is sick and worried. Perceiving the physician as busy and under pressure, the patient may feel like an intruder. The doctor is often brusque, does not take the time to listen, neglects to explain. His prognosis may be discouraging, his therapy prolonged and unpleasant. He charges a lot, earns more, and lives better than the patient, perhaps causing irritation and envy. Some patients are just plain frightened away from reputable doctors whose rapport falls below that which quacks are able to muster. Even patients who think well of their own doctors may think ill of doctors as a group. The power side of establishment medicine has alienated many people. Organized medicine, they have felt, works for its own economic and political self-interest more than for the common good. Such an image helps quackery. For throughout history, any criticism of the power or the science of orthodox medicine has been pounced upon by the quack, magnified, and loudly trumpeted abroad.

The Quack

The unorthodox healer does not need to observe the restraints of reputable medicine. Where true medical science is complex, the quack can oversimplify. All diseases are catarrh, and Peruna cures catarrh. Where ailments are self-limiting, the quack makes nature his secret ally, crediting his tonic with curing tuberculosis when in fact nature has alleviated postnasal drip. Where the placebo effect may operate, the quack prescribes it adeptly. It may be something for arthritis as ancient as a copper bracelet or as modern as "moon dust."

The quack pays more attention to the person than to the ailment, seeking to convince the patient that the treatment is necessary. A dose of fright can be an effective persuader. Ralph Lee Smith, in his book *At Your Own Risk,* tells of infiltrating a school run by a Texas chiropractor aimed at teaching other chiropractors how to increase their incomes. *"If the patient has a pain in his left shoulder,"* the professor said, his pupils should ask, *"Has the pain started in your right shoulder yet?"* [The so-called "Yet Disease."]

Along with fright goes tenderness. The quack manages a superb bedside manner. Since he can't really provide a cure if major disease is present, he specializes in promises, sympathy, consideration and concern. The patient responds to this attention. This helps explain one of the odd paradoxes relating to quackery—that failure seldom diminishes patient loyalty. When regulatory agencies seek to prosecute quacks, the agencies have a difficult task getting hapless patients to testify in court. Partly this results from the desire to avoid public exposure as a dupe. But more of this objection to testifying rests on an inability to realize that deception has taken place. The quack has done such a good job of exuding sincerity that his explanations seem all too plausible. Even patients faced with death believe in the "kindly" man who says his remedy would have worked if treatment had only begun a little sooner.

Some points I have been making suggest that doctors might improve their human relationships. Other aspects of vulnerability may be so inherent in human nature that they can never be eliminated. While the physician seeks to help his patient if he can, he must sometimes confess that he cannot. The quack need make no such confession, for honesty is not contained in his code of ethics. This gives the charlatan great advantage in competing with the physician for the kind of patient I have described. For the quack can promise anything— tailoring his appeals to all the susceptibilities, vulnerabilities, and curiosities which human nature reveals.

What of the Future?

Efforts to educate against the dangers of quackery have met with only modest success. Efforts to control quackery by law have done somewhat better. The Food and Drug Administration and the Postal Service have driven many misleading and fraudulent drugs and devices from the marketplace and have put some charlatans in jail. The Kefauver-Harris Act of 1962 requires that new drugs be proven effective before they can be marketed. As a result of this, it seems unlikely that any new worthless cancer treatment will reach the national peak achieved in their heyday by Harry Hoxsey's weird concoction and by Krebiozen. Still, regulators keep busy with other important tasks, their appropriations are perennially inadequate, legal procedures take years to reach fruition, penalties are seldom heavy, state laws are generally weak, and some foreign countries permit quack promotions outlawed in our nation. In view of this, as well as the quack's agility and the customer's eagerness, legal controls hardly seem likely to eradicate charlatanism.

Indeed, during the last few years, I have wondered if quackery's future has not brightened, because so many young people have assumed a neo-romantic posture that makes them highly vulnerable. They have become skeptical of gigantic institutions, including big science, and look askance at reason as a way for seeking truth. Whatever merit may lie in suspecting reason's inadequacies, the reaction has often gone to the extreme of deliberate flirtation, if not liaison, with wild varieties of unreason. Astrology has soared, not as a pastime, but for real. Publishing houses have minted millions from it, while almost every college campus has a peripheral course in "reading the stars." Spiritualism has made a comeback, with "spiritual churches" blossoming in almost every city. Tarot cards, palmistry, and numerology have flourished. Paperbacks on these themes have been among the hottest items in university bookstores from Cambridge to Berkeley. Witchcraft and devil worship have made an appearance. Many among the young have turned their backs on civilization and its discontents, sometimes retreating into communes remotely located, sometimes merely buying "organic" foods at the nearest health food store.

One may strongly sympathize, I hope, with sensitive youth's criticisms of the disorders of our world. But those who embrace irrationality so fervently furnish a fertile recruiting ground for unscientific health wares.

For, as we have seen, quacks are agile. They sense quickly and rush in to exploit people's real concerns. Thus, for many timeless reasons and for new reasons too, health quackery may be expected to continue. Despite the gloomy prospects, both education and regulation must be employed vigorously to restrain as much as possible quackery's toll in wasted resources and human suffering.

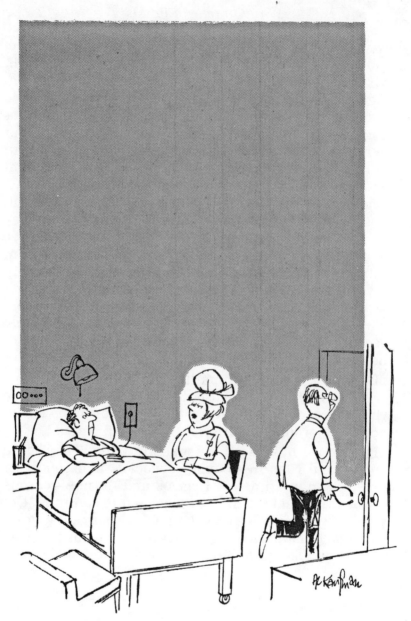

"Touchy, isn't he? Just because I corrected his diagnosis."

GETTING THE MOST FROM YOUR DOCTOR

*Good medical care is a partnership
between you and your doctor.*

BY

PHILIP R. ALPER, M.D.
*Assistant Clinical Professor of Medicine
University of California Medical School*

Unless he is Marcus Welby, your doctor will treat more than one patient per week. He may not be able to answer all your questions or solve all your problems. He may get tired or irritable, rushed or preoccupied. He may keep you waiting. And he will sometimes make mistakes.

But don't despair. In most parts of this country, good medical care can be yours if you work at two things— finding a doctor you can trust and learning to communicate with him.

Your Doctor's Personality

Some years ago, an eloquent Texan named Max Scheid told a medical audience what he expected from his physician:

—Honesty.
—Care for myself and family in sickness and in health.
—Treatment as an individual with dignity from the doctor and also his staff.
—Availability when needed.
—Concern for soul as well as body.
—Treatment on the adult level.
—A charge of a customary fee.
—Use of an accredited hospital.
—Personal concern with the patient's health.
—Referral to a competent physician when necessary.
—The ability to listen as well as trust.
—Ordering only the necessary laboratory tests.
—A non-defensive practice of medicine.
—Prayer for the patient.

After Mr. Scheid had finished, his doctor spoke. A warm and personal relationship existed between the two, and the doctor acknowledged this with visible pleasure.

Contrast this with auto-magnate Henry Ford II's expectation of medical care as reported in *Medical Economics* magazine. Mr. Ford wanted top-flight doctors who worked in top-flight institutions. He wasn't interested in personalities, but just in getting the job done quickly and efficiently. His expectations were all *technical* rather than *personal* or even a mixture of both. In fact, they bore a startling resemblance to automobile repair!

Obviously, these two gentlemen look at medical care differently. Mr. Scheid sees his physician as a part of his life. Mr. Ford views his as a periodic and barely tolerable intruder into his busy schedule.

Primary Care

For first-rate care to occur, your personality and your doctor's personality must fit one another. This is especially true for so-called *primary care*—ongoing care by a doctor who knows you and is the first one you turn to for help.

Some people are more comfortable with an *institution* than with a particular physician. They may be perfectly content to be seen episodically on an out-patient basis or in emergency rooms by any number of different physicians. This is far from ideal care, but it is common in county hospitals and in some group practices such as the Kaiser-Permanente clinics and hospitals. I call this *compromise care*. With luck, a strong constitution and a basically good medical staff, it may work out.

It is far better to choose a *personal physician*. He or she may be in either solo or group private practice or in a multi-doctor clinic. Even in a group, a personal physician ally can help steer you through the medical maze while looking out for your welfare. Most groups, including the large ones, allow patients to pick a physician from their roster.

329

Choosing A Doctor

Your best bet is a specialist who is board-certified in internal medicine or family practice. Such a physician is sure to have taken advanced training in the diagnosis and treatment of general medical problems.

Staff affiliation with a hospital connected with a medical school indicates that a physician is working with up-to-date colleagues and is apt to be one himself. Affiliation with a hospital that trains interns and residents is also favorable. Less certain is affiliation with only proprietary hospitals—especially small ones—unless they are the only ones in the area. Lack of any hospital affiliation should be suspect.

Consumer-oriented directories which list a doctor's affiliations and credentials are appearing lately. But much, if not all, of the information they contain can readily be obtained by calling the doctor's office, his hospital and the county medical society.

Other positive indicators include membership in the American College of Physicians or the American College of Surgeons (though a surgeon is not a usual choice for a primary physician). Teaching appointments in a medical school are also a good sign.

Consumerist Ralph Nader favors physicians who practice in a group rather than alone. His theory is that in a group, since doctors can watch each other, frank incompetence is less likely to occur. Although this theory has considerable merit, membership in a group is no guarantee against mediocrity. Besides, there are many outstanding solo physicians. In 1974 the American Board of Internal Medicine offered a voluntary "recertification" exam which was taken by 4,000 doctors. This detailed test probed knowledge across a broad range of medical topics. The Board expected that physicians practicing in universities would rank highest, followed by doctors in group practice and with solo doctors trailing badly. However, the results showed little difference among the three physician categories.

My own bias is toward a well-credentialed, well-affiliated, solo physician or one practicing in a group *in the same specialty*. Should you need referral to a specialist, a first-class primary physician is likely to select a specialist of equal caliber. The defect of multispecialty groups is lack of free choice of consultants. Then again, some of these specialty groups are outstanding across the board from specialty to specialty. The Palo Alto and Mayo Clinics are examples. Some people use multispecialty groups for some of their medical care and go outside them for particular problems.

Asking a neighbor, fellow worker or relative for the name of a doctor is an exceedingly common practice, but is often criticized as unreliable. If people do it, though, there has to be a reason. Perhaps they don't know any better way. If so, the suggestions given above should help. Nonetheless, non-doctors are not entirely lacking in judgment when it comes to evaluating physicians. It doesn't take an expert to evaluate courtesy, attentiveness, whether an office is efficiently run or whether the doctor is personable and likely to get along with you. So personal recommendations *do* have a place—but a limited one.

Meeting Your Doctor

An excellent way to begin your relationship with a new doctor is a thorough physical examination when you are not ill. Such an examination will give your doctor a "baseline"—a personal health profile against which he can compare any changes in future years. This can be a big help in making a diagnosis and planning treatment later on.

A "get-acquainted" physical exam is also an ideal

time to bring up any health questions which have been troubling you. "My father had diabetes. What are my chances of getting it?" Or perhaps, "What do you think of vasectomies?" Questions like these are important, but tend to be put aside during the treatment of an acute illness.

If you do not wish to have a complete physical exam, it still may pay to schedule a brief visit with your prospective doctor. Meeting him should help you decide whether he is the person you wish to consult in the future. During this visit you can also sign a release form which your new doctor can use to obtain your past medical records.

Advance "registration" has an additional advantage. Some doctors will not accept new patients under emergency conditions, particularly outside of regular office hours. Once a doctor has accepted you as a patient, however, he has a *legal* obligation either to treat you or to provide a substitute.

Having chosen a primary physician, try to learn his routine. Some doctors have printed instruction sheets for this purpose. If yours does not, ask questions. Which is his day off? Who will cover for him in his absence? Does he make house calls? Which hospital does he use? This last bit of information is especially important. Few physicians are on the staff of every hospital in town. In an emergency, ambulance drivers usually take patients to the nearest hospital—unless they are told differently. If you go to the wrong hospital, your doctor may not be able to take care of you.

Telephone Manners

Proper use of the telephone can do a lot to make your doctor's life easier while helping you at the same time to receive better service. Before you call his office, take a moment to organize your thoughts. What is bothering you? When did it begin? If you have a pain, does it come and go or is it steady? Does anything bring it on or relieve it? If you have an infection or any other reason to suspect you might have a fever, take your temperature.

Try to decide whether your problem is urgent or not. You are not expected to know all the answers, but often you will have a good idea. For example, a cold lingering on for five days is not an emergency, but squeezing chest pain may be. If in doubt, simply say, "I am not sure if this is urgent, but . . ."

It is not unusual for a busy physician to receive 50–100 telephone calls per day—many more than he could possibly handle by himself. So when you call, don't start out by asking to speak with him. His receptionist or nurse is trained to assemble the information needed for a preliminary evaluation of your situation. She is an *extension* of your doctor and will usually know which matters she can handle by herself and which ones the doctor must handle personally. After she is finished, if you still feel you must speak with the doctor, that is the time to ask.

When you telephone, have a pad and pencil handy to write down any instructions you receive. Memory is notoriously faulty. Call as early in the day as possible. That way your doctor can handle your case most efficiently—while his assistants are on duty to help him and while hospitals and laboratories are able to give their best services. Above all, avoid waiting until Friday afternoon for a problem which has troubled you all week!

When you call to ask for a prescription refill, know the phone number of your drugstore. Make your request during the doctor's office hours and before you get down to the last pill. That way the doctor can review your office record to see whether you still need the medication, whether the dosage should be changed, and so on. Such a review will make your medical care safer. If you telephone outside of office hours, many physicians (especially those covering another doctor's practice) will order only enough medication for a few days. That is the safest way in the absence of your medical records, but it does increase the cost of your medication.

In an emergency, try to telephone your doctor immediately. Don't just show up in a hospital emergency room. Advance notice to your doctor will enable him to alert the emergency room personnel so that they may begin treatment or arrange for tests that he wants. Also, it is very exasperating for a doctor to have a patient arrive at an emergency room moments after he has finished treating another patient and left the hospital.

Talking With Your Doctor

Although good communication is essential to good medical care, speaking with a doctor is not always easy. You may be afraid (*What will he tell me? Maybe the worst is true?*) Or embarrassed (*I can't admit that. What will he think?*) Or even resentful (*Who does he think he is? He probably won't even be able to help me.*)

Try not to let feelings like these create a barrier between you and your doctor. Instead, put the feelings to work *for* you by sharing them with him. State your prejudices and concerns such as "I don't like to take medicines." Or "I don't want to take anything that might do me more harm than good." Or perhaps "I had some bad reactions to medication in the past." You may have heard or read something or seen something on TV that strikes you as relevant to your condition. If any of these—or other things—are on your mind, be sure to mention them.

334

Suppose you have doubts about a recommended treatment. Voice them. Don't play a waiting game and end up with a misunderstanding which could have been avoided. Relating to a physician should not mean taking a back seat. Doctors know that how a patient feels about his treatment may influence its outcome. If you find a treatment particularly objectionable, your doctor may suggest a more acceptable alternative. Even if you are slated to disagree (let's say you think your heart condition would best be treated by vitamins rather than digitalis), you still owe it to yourself to hear the doctor's point of view. Approached properly, a compromise satisfactory to both you and your doctor may be possible.

Ask Questions

Doctors may sometimes be authoritarian and even patronizing. It is an occupational hazard—the result of years of counseling and treating others. Don't accept this! Ask your physician to explain *why* you are having your symptoms. Why, for example, your ulcer hurts, and why it hurts less if you drink milk. Ask what the medication he suggests is supposed to do. What will happen if the condition remains untreated. Whether there are alternative treatments. The key word is *ask*. The more you know, the more you can help yourself and help the doctor to help you.

Make sure your doctor's explanations make sense to you. Even very technical concepts can be phrased in words that are easy for non-doctors to understand. For example, why does a "spastic stomach" hurt? There are a number of explanations, but a simple analogy can make the point. Clench your fist as tightly as you can for five or ten minutes. Not only will your hand hurt, but it will get stiff and be difficult to open. In other words, the muscles go into spasm. The logic of using a drug to reduce the spasm is then obvious. Similarly, if you are tense, you can actually feel the tension in the muscles of your face or arms. It is not difficult to imagine the same thing happening inside of you. Perhaps a medication to relieve tension is in order. Or perhaps only a change in your routine. Knowing the cause of your problem is sometimes enough to relieve it.

Learn the names of your medications. Ask about their side effects a.id whether treatment should be stopped when you feel better or continued beyond that point. Continuing medication is especially important in painless but potentially serious conditions such as high blood pressure. Untreated, hypertension can lead to heart attacks and strokes. Patients who do not understand why they need long-term treatment often discontinue their medications and then develop complications. Lack of understanding may not be the only problem, however. Unpleasant side effects (dry mouth, stuffy nose or other uncomfortable effects of the drugs apart from their basic treatment function) may occur. If you suffer side effects, don't simply stop your medicine. Discuss them with your doctor. Often a change of dose or medicine can be worked out to your advantage.

If You Have A Grievance

As in any human relationship, miscommunications between doctor and patient are inevitable from time to time. Not long ago, I heard about a patient who left another physician "because he was cold." I was astonished, since this particular physician cared very much about his patients and I knew him to be a very warm human being. What actually had happened? The lady had a lengthy list of puzzling complaints. The doctor was concentrating intently on what she was saying, trying to organize her symptoms into a pattern that would lead to a diagnosis. His effort must have shown on his face—but the *meaning* of his expression was misinterpreted as coldness.

The lesson is clear. Don't be too hasty to judge. If you have a grievance, *voice it*. "You don't seem to care, doctor." Or, "I am not sure you are listening to me." Whatever. Perhaps the doctor really is listening. Or maybe he is tired or preoccupied with another patient's problem—or even one of his own. The doctor *himself* should appreciate being told that you are displeased so that he can either straighten out your misconception or apologize if he is in the wrong. (If he can't take such criticism, then you know he isn't the doctor for you.) Don't suffer in silence or leave the doctor's care without telling him why.

Language can cause problems too. Physicians often choose their words poorly when trying to reassure patients about minor but irritating symptoms. When a doctor says, "It's nothing," he probably means, "I think it isn't serious and should clear up by itself with time." When a doctor says, "It's your nerves," he is probably trying to say "It's your body's reaction to tension." But to some patients, such remarks may sound like an accusation that they are imagining or exaggerating their symptoms. Medical school does not turn doctors into linguists. (Quite the contrary.) If a doctor's clumsy shorthand remarks bother you—say so and ask for a fuller explanation. I would caution, however, that not every ailment warrants a lengthy explanation or an intensive series of diagnostic tests right away. Most illnesses are self-limiting. So be prepared to accept an answer like, "If your problem does not clear up in the near future, we can explore it further."

While preparing this chapter, I took an informal poll among physician colleagues. The need for patients to voice their grievances was a recurrent theme. A typical comment: "If you have a problem with a doctor—his office, his bills, *or him*—let him know. He'll appreciate it and try to help." Resolving disagreements and dissatisfactions can do much to build bonds between human beings. Consultation or a change of doctors will always be possible. You'd be surprised, however, how often a strong mutual understanding can develop in spite of some initial friction. Two quick illustrations will show how this works.

Dr. X was attending a man who was having a third operation to salvage a knee which was badly damaged by arthritis. One day, as the doctor was about to leave the hospital room, the patient asked him to sit down. "I wouldn't tell you this if I didn't like you and feel that you would want to know," said the patient with masterful tact. "But you are in and out of here like a flash. Some patients would get the idea that you are only interested in rushing around to make more money."

Dr. X was shocked. There were many excuses— emergency calls, hospital committee work, and the like. But as he thought about it, the doctor realized that although he himself handled only the patient's non-surgical care, the man's bad luck with surgery frustrated and bothered the doctor so much that he cut his visits short. Instead of offering excuses, Dr. X told the truth. The exchange cleared the air and solved the problem.

The other incident involved a healthy woman who had been checked routinely by Dr. Y for many years. He knew her and her family well. On the morning of her appointment, three unscheduled patients arrived one after another with urgent problems. Normally, Dr. Y was able to stick to his schedule well, so the woman was waiting patiently. When the third emergency patient was taken, the doctor's nurse told her that there would be an additional delay. Rather than wait any longer, the patient scheduled a new appointment. But instead of keeping it, she sent a request to Dr. Y to transfer her records to another physician.

Dr. Y might simply have complied, but the incident didn't sit right with him. So he telephoned the patient's husband. The patient was upset about both having to relieve her daughter who was covering her job and "seeing three people who came in after me go in first—especially after ten years as a patient." After explaining the circumstances to the husband, Dr. Y added his hope that the relationship would not end on a sour note. "I would be happy to speak to your wife if she would like to call," he concluded.

Shortly afterward, the patient did call. She had a point. The nurse could have told her earlier about the additional delay. But the doctor had a point too. "You have been lucky never to have had an emergency yourself," he said, "but if you had, *you* would have bumped the schedule and someone else would have been unhappy." The conversation ended pleasantly, and the appointment was rescheduled.

Remember, good medical care should be a partnership, with open two-way communication between you and your doctor. Like most things in life, it is available to those who work for it.

A FINAL COMMENT

Nobody likes to think of himself as someone who would go to a quack. Yet quackery is thriving. *The Health Robbers* was written to protect you from being a victim. Our fond hope is that it will also arouse you to press for stronger consumer protection laws and better health education.

In matters of health there should be no tolerance for deception.

—*The Lehigh Valley Committee*
Against Health Fraud, Inc.